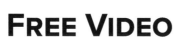 **FREE VIDEO**  **FREE VIDEO**

Essential Test Tips Video from Trivium Test Prep!

Dear Customer,

Thank you for purchasing from Trivium Test Prep! We're honored to help you prepare for your CEN exam.

To show our appreciation, we're offering a **FREE *CEN Essential Test Tips* Video by Trivium Test Prep**.* Our video includes 35 test preparation strategies that will make you successful on the CEN. All we ask is that you email us your feedback and describe your experience with our product. Amazing, awful, or just so-so: we want to hear what you have to say!

To receive your **FREE *CEN Essential Test Tips* Video**, please email us at 5star@ triviumtestprep.com. Include "Free 5 Star" in the subject line and the following information in your email:

1. The title of the product you purchased.

2. Your rating from 1 – 5 (with 5 being the best).

3. Your feedback about the product, including how our materials helped you meet your goals and ways in which we can improve our products.

4. Your full name and shipping address so we can send your **FREE *CEN Essential Test Tips* Video**.

If you have any questions or concerns please feel free to contact us directly at 5star@ triviumtestprep.com.

Thank you!

- Trivium Test Prep Team

*To get access to the free video please email us at 5star@triviumtestprep.com, and please follow the instructions above.

CEN STUDY GUIDE

Review Book with Practice Test Questions for the
Certified Emergency Nurse Exam

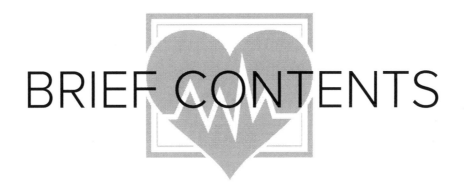

BRIEF CONTENTS

TABLE OF CONTENTS

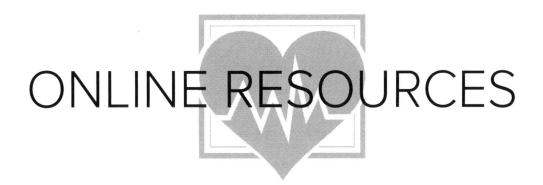

ONLINE RESOURCES

To help you fully prepare for your CEN exam, Trivium includes online resources with the purchase of this study guide.

Practice Test

In addition to the practice test included in this book, we also offer an online exam. Since many exams today are computer based, getting to practice your test-taking skills on the computer is a great way to prepare.

Flash Cards

A convenient supplement to this study guide, Trivium's flash cards enable you to review important terms easily on your computer or smartphone.

Cheat Sheets

Review the core skills you need to master the exam with easy-to-read Cheat Sheets.

From Stress to Success

Watch From Stress to Success, a brief but insightful YouTube video that offers the tips, tricks, and secrets experts use to score higher on the exam.

Reviews

Leave a review, send us helpful feedback, or sign up for Trivium promotions—including free books!

Access these materials at: **www.triviumtestprep.com/cen-online-resources**

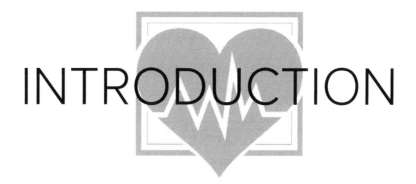

INTRODUCTION

Congratulations on choosing to take the Certified Emergency Nurse (CEN) Exam! Passing the CEN is an important step forward in your nursing career.

In the following pages, you will find information about the CEN, what to expect on test day, how to use this book, and the content covered on the exam. We also encourage you to visit the website of the Board of Certification for Emergency Nursing (https://bcen.org) to register for the exam and find the most current information on the CEN.

THE BCEN CERTIFICATION PROCESS

The **CERTIFIED EMERGENCY NURSE (CEN) EXAM** is developed by the Board of Certification for Emergency Nursing (BCEN) as part of its certification program for emergency nurses. To qualify for the exam, you must have a current Registered Nurse license in the United States or its territories. No experience is required to qualify for the exam, but the BCEN recommends that you have worked for at least two years in the emergency department.

To register for the exam, you must first apply through the BCEN website (https://bcen.org/cen/apply-schedule). After your application is accepted, you will receive an email with instructions on how to register for the exam. The CEN is administered at Pearson VUE testing centers around the nation.

Once you have met the qualifications and passed the exam, you will have your CEN certification, and you may use the credentials as long as your certification is valid. You will need to recertify every four years.

CEN QUESTIONS AND TIMING

The CEN consists of **175 QUESTIONS**. Only 150 of these questions are scored; 25 are unscored, or pretest questions. These questions are included by the BCEN to test their suitability for inclusion in future tests. You'll have no way of knowing which questions are unscored, so treat every question like it counts.

The questions on the CEN are multiple-choice with four answer choices. Some questions will include exhibits such as ECG reading strips or laboratory results. The CEN has no guess penalty, so you should always guess if you do not know the answer to a question.

You will have **3 HOURS** to complete the test. You may take breaks at any point during the exam, but you will not be given extra time.

CEN CONTENT AREAS

The BCEN framework is broken down into seven sections loosely based on human body systems and one section devoted to professional issues. The table below gives the breakdown of the questions on the exam. (The detailed outline for each section is given in the relevant chapter.)

Summary of CEN Content Outline		
	SECTION	APPROX. NO. OF QUESTIONS
1.	Cardiovascular Emergencies	23
2.	Respiratory Emergencies	19
3.	Neurological Emergencies	19
4.	Gastrointestinal, Genitourinary, Gynecology, and Obstetrical Emergencies	24
5.	Psychosocial and Medical Emergencies	29
6.	Maxillofacial, Ocular, Orthopedic, and Wound Emergencies	24
7.	Environment and Toxicology Emergencies, and Communicable Diseases	18
8.	Professional Issues	19
Total		**175 questions**

EXAM RESULTS

Once you have completed your test, the staff at the Pearson VUE testing center will give you a score report; you can also request to receive the report via email. The score report will include your raw score (the number of questions you answered correctly) for the whole test and for each content area.

The report will also include a pass/fail designation. The number of correct answers needed to pass the exam will vary slightly depending on the questions included in your version of the test (i.e., if you took a version of the test with harder questions, the passing score will be lower). For most test takers, a passing score will be between 105 and 110 questions answered correctly.

If you do not pass the exam, you will be able to reapply and retake the test after 90 days.

USING THIS BOOK

This book is divided into two sections. In the content area review, you will find the pathophysiology, diagnostic findings, and treatment protocols for the conditions included in the CEN framework. Throughout the chapter you'll also see Quick Review Questions that will help reinforce important concepts and skills.

The book also includes two full-length practice tests (one in the book and one online) with answer rationales. You can use these tests to gauge your readiness for the test and determine which content areas you may need to review more thoroughly.

ASCENCIA TEST PREP

With health care fields such as nursing, pharmacy, emergency care, and physical therapy becoming the fastest-growing industries in the United States, individuals looking to enter the health care industry or rise in their field need high-quality, reliable resources. Ascencia Test Prep's study guides and test preparation materials are developed by credentialed industry professionals with years of experience in their respective fields. Ascencia recognizes that health care professionals nurture bodies and spirits, and save lives. Ascencia Test Prep's mission is to help health care workers grow.

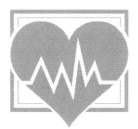

CARDIOVASCULAR EMERGENCIES

BCEN CONTENT OUTLINE

* **A. ACUTE CORONARY SYNDROME**
  B. Aneurysm/dissection
* **C. CARDIOPULMONARY ARREST**
* **D. DYSRHYTHMIAS**
  E. Endocarditis
* **F. HEART FAILURE**
  G. Hypertension
  H. Pericardial tamponade
  I. Pericarditis
  J. Peripheral vascular disease (e.g., arterial, venous)
  K. Thromboembolic disease (e.g., deep vein thrombosis [DVT])
  L. Trauma
* **M. SHOCK (CARDIOGENIC AND OBSTRUCTIVE)**

ACUTE CORONARY SYNDROME (ACS)   ✱

PATHOPHYSIOLOGY

ACUTE CORONARY SYNDROME (ACS) is an umbrella term for cardiac conditions in which thrombosis impairs blood flow in coronary arteries. ANGINA PECTORIS (commonly just called angina) is chest pain caused by narrowed coronary arteries and presents with negative troponin, an ST depression, and T wave changes.

- **STABLE ANGINA** usually resolves in about 5 minutes, is resolved with medications or with rest, and can be triggered by exertion, large meals, and extremely hot or cold temperatures.

- **UNSTABLE ANGINA** can occur at any time and typically lasts longer (> 20 minutes). The pain is usually rated as more severe than stable angina and is not easily relieved by the administration of nitrates.
- **VARIANT ANGINA** (also called Prinzmetal angina or vasospastic angina) is episodes of angina and temporary ST elevation caused by spasms in the coronary artery. Chest pain is easily relieved by nitrates.

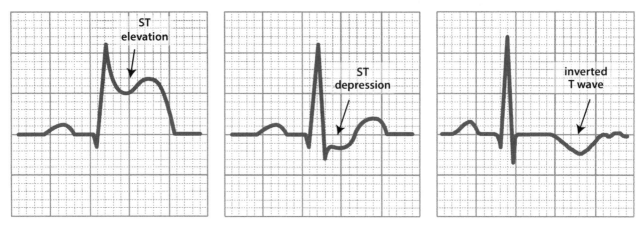

Figure 1.1. ECG Changes Associated with ACS

A **MYOCARDIAL INFARCTION (MI)**, or ischemia of the heart muscle, occurs when the coronary arteries are partly or completely occluded. MI is diagnosed via positive troponin and ECG changes; it is classified by the behavior of the ST wave. A **NON-ST-ELEVATION MYOCARDIAL INFARCTION (NSTEMI)** includes an ST depression and a T wave inversion. An **ST-ELEVATION MYOCARDIAL INFARCTION (STEMI)** includes an elevated ST (> 1 mm), indicating a complete occlusion of a coronary artery. Signs, symptoms, and diagnostic findings for MI vary depending on which coronary artery is occluded (see Table 1.1 below).

HELPFUL HINT

Papillary muscle rupture is a rare but serious complication that occurs 2 – 8 days post MI. Patients will present with hemodynamic compromise; pulmonary edema, new, loud systolic murmur; and a large V wave in PAOP. Papillary muscle rupture usually requires immediate surgical repair.

Table 1.1. ECG Changes Seen in MI by Location		
LOCATION	**DESCRIPTION**	**ST CHANGES**
anterior-wall MI	occlusion of the LAD artery, which supplies blood to the anterior of the left atrium and ventricle	ST changes in V1 – V4
inferior-wall MI	occlusion of the RCA, which supplies blood to the right atrium and ventricle, the SA node, and the AV node	ST changes in II, III, aVF
right ventricular infarction	may occur with inferior-wall MI	ST changes in V4R – V6R
lateral-wall MI	occlusion of the left circumflex artery, which supplies blood to the left atrium and the posterior/lateral walls of the left ventricle	ST changes may be seen in I, aVL, V5, or V6
posterior-wall MI	occlusion of the RCA or left circumflex artery	ST elevation in V7 – V9 and ST depression in V1 – V4

DIAGNOSIS

- continuous chest pain that may radiate to the back, arm, or jaw (possible Levine's sign)

- upper abdominal pain (more common in adults > 65, people with diabetes, and females)

- dyspnea

- nausea or vomiting

- dizziness or syncope

- diaphoresis and pallor

- palpitations

- elevated troponin (> 0.01 ng/mL)

- elevated CK-MB (> 2.5%)

MANAGEMENT

- 160 – 325 mg aspirin (chewed and swallowed); clopidogrel for patients who cannot take aspirin

- NSTEMI: initially treated with medication
  - ☐ nitroglycerin for vasodilatation of coronary arteries
  - ☐ beta blockers or calcium channel blockers to reduce myocardial oxygen demand
  - ☐ heparin to improve blood flow
  - ☐ morphine if pain is not relieved by nitroglycerin

- STEMI: immediate fibrinolytic therapy or PCI
  - ☐ goal for door to balloon time: 90 minutes
  - ☐ goal for door to fibrinolytic therapy: 30 minutes

QUICK REVIEW QUESTION

1. A patient with a new complaint of chest pain and left arm pain is found clutching his chest. He is in bed and appears pale and diaphoretic. His heart rate is 55 bpm. What priority interventions should the cardiac nurse take?

ANEURYSM/DISSECTION

PATHOPHYSIOLOGY

An AORTIC RUPTURE, a complete tear in the wall of the aorta, rapidly leads to hemorrhagic shock and death. An AORTIC DISSECTION is a tear in the aortic intima; the tear allows blood to enter the aortic media. Both aortic rupture and dissection will lead to hemorrhagic shock and death without immediate intervention.

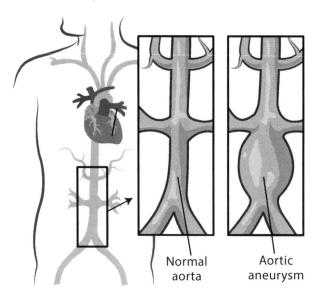

Figure 1.2. Abdominal Aortic Aneurysm (AAA)

DIAGNOSIS

- sharp, severe pain in the chest, back, abdomen, or flank; often described as "tearing"
- rapid, weak, or absent pulse
- a blood pressure difference of ≥ 20 mm Hg between the left and right arms
- new-onset murmur
- diaphoresis and pallor
- nausea and vomiting
- hypotension
- orthopnea
- CT scan, transesophageal echocardiogram (TEE), angiogram, or chest MRI

TREATMENT AND MANAGEMENT

HELPFUL HINT
Positive inotropes are contraindicated in patients with aortic dissection because the medications increase stress on the aortic wall.

- pain management (usually morphine)
- beta blockers; nitroprusside may also be given
- hemodynamically unstable patients: immediate surgical repair usually required

QUICK REVIEW QUESTION

2. A patient reports new-onset, sharp pain and describes it as tearing. The blood pressure in the right arm is 85/62 mm Hg. What should the nurse do next?

DYSRHYTHMIAS AND CONDUCTION DEFECTS

A cardiac DYSRHYTHMIA is an abnormal heartbeat or rhythm. Treatment is based on whether the patient is deemed hemodynamically stable or unstable.

- stable patients: noninvasive interventions or drugs to correct an abnormal rhythm

- unstable patients: appropriate electrical therapy

HELPFUL HINT

When treating dysrhythmias, medical staff should always consider a hypotensive patient unstable.

Bradycardia ✷

PATHOPHYSIOLOGY

BRADYCARDIA is a heart rate of < 60 bpm. It results from a decrease in the sinus node impulse formation (automaticity). Bradycardia is normal in certain individuals and does not require an intervention if the patient is stable. Symptomatic patients, however, need immediate treatment to address the cause of bradycardia and to correct the dysrhythmia. Symptoms of bradycardia may include hypotension, syncope, confusion, or dyspnea.

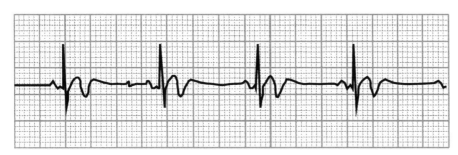

Figure 1.3. ECG: Bradycardia

MANAGEMENT

- asymptomatic, stable patients
    - ☐ no intervention required; may be monitored for development of symptoms
- symptomatic, hemodynamically stable patients
    - ☐ monitor while determining underlying cause
- symptomatic, hemodynamically unstable patients
    - ☐ first line: atropine 0.5 mg for first dose, with a maximum of 3 mg total
    - ☐ second line: dopamine or epinephrine if atropine is ineffective or if maximum dose of atropine already given
    - ☐ refractory bradycardia: TCP

3. A patient presents with complaints of confusion, dizziness, and dyspnea. The patient's blood pressure is 72/40 mm Hg, with a heart rate of 32 bpm and O$_2$ saturation of 92% on room air. What priority intervention should the nurse prepare for?

★ Narrow-Complex Tachycardias

PATHOPHYSIOLOGY

NARROW-COMPLEX TACHYCARDIAS (also called SUPRAVENTRICULAR TACHYCARDIA [**SVT**]) are dysrhythmias with > 100 bpm and a narrow QRS complex (< 0.12 seconds). The dysrhythmia originates at or above the bundle of His (supraventricular), resulting in rapid ventricular activation. Narrow-complex tachycardias are often asymptomatic. Symptomatic patients may have palpitations, chest pain, hypotension, and dyspnea.

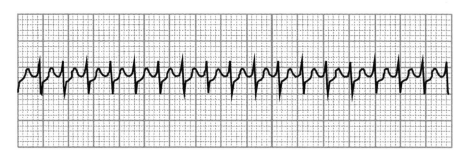

Figure 1.4. Supraventricular Tachycardia

MANAGEMENT

- first line treatment: vagal maneuvers
- second line treatment
  - rapid bolus dose of adenosine (6 mg) to restore sinus rhythm if dysrhythmia continues
  - second dose (this time 12 mg) may be administered if chemical cardioversion does not occur within 1 – 2 minutes
- refractory SVT
  - stable patients: calcium channel blockers, beta blockers, or digoxin may also be given
  - unstable patients and patients for whom medications are ineffective: synchronized cardioversion

QUICK REVIEW QUESTION

4. A patient in SVT is unresponsive to vagal maneuvers. What intervention is likely to be ordered next?

Atrial Fibrillation and Flutter

PATHOPHYSIOLOGY

ATRIAL FIBRILLATION (A-FIB) is an irregular narrow-complex tachycardia. During A-fib, the heart cannot adequately empty, causing blood to pool and clots to form, increasing stroke risk. The irregular atrial contractions also decrease cardiac output (CO). The ECG in A-fib will show an irregular rhythm with no P waves and an undeterminable atrial rate (Figure 1.5).

HELPFUL HINT

A-fib is the most common cardiac dysrhythmia. It occurs in approximately 2 – 6 million individuals in the United States annually.

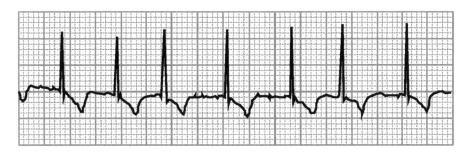

Figure 1.5. ECG: Atrial Fibrillation (A-fib)

During ATRIAL FLUTTER, the atria beat regularly but too fast (240 – 400 bpm), causing multiple atrial beats in between the ventricular beat. Atrial flutter can be regular or irregular. The ECG in atrial flutter will show a saw-toothed flutter and multiple P waves for each QRS complex (Figure 1.6).

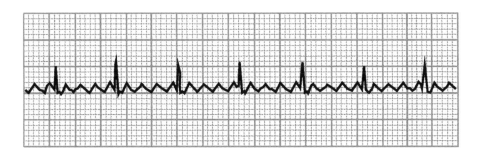

Figure 1.6. ECG: Atrial Flutter

MANAGEMENT

- adenosine: slows the rhythm so that it may be identified, but will not convert dysrhythmia to a sinus rhythm
- hemodynamically stable patients
    - calcium channel blockers, beta blockers, or cardiac glycoside to slow the rhythm
    - antidysrhythmics may be administered to convert to sinus rhythm
- hemodynamically unstable patients: cardioversion required
- anticoagulants to lower risk of stroke
- cardiac ablation may be used to correct A-fib and atrial flutter

5. A patient presents with A-fib. Vital signs are as follows:

BP	125/80 mm Hg
HR	150 bpm
RR	23

What intervention should the nurse anticipate?

★ Ventricular Tachycardia and Fibrillation

PATHOPHYSIOLOGY

HELPFUL HINT

Torsades de pointes, a type of V-tach with irregular QRS complexes, occurs with a prolonged QT interval. It can be congenital or caused by antidysrhythmics, antipsychotics, hypokalemia, or hypomagnesemia.

VENTRICULAR TACHYCARDIA (**V-TACH**) is tachycardia originating below the bundle of His, resulting in slowed ventricular activation. During V-tach, ≥ 3 consecutive ventricular beats occur at a rate > 100 bpm. V-tach is often referred to as a WIDE-COMPLEX TACHYCARDIA because of the width of the QRS complex.

Because the ventricles cannot refill before contracting, patients in this rhythm may have reduced CO, resulting in hypotension. V-tach may be short and asymptomatic, or it may precede V-fib and cardiac arrest.

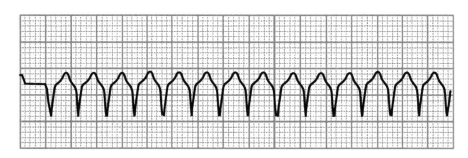

Figure 1.7. ECG: Monomorphic Ventricular Tachycardia (V-tach)

During VENTRICULAR FIBRILLATION (**V-FIB**) the ventricles contract rapidly (300 – 400 bpm) with no organized rhythm. There is no CO. The ECG will initially show COARSE **V-FIB** with an amplitude > 3 mm (Figure 1.8). As V-fib continues, the amplitude of the waveform decreases, progressing through FINE **V-FIB** (< 3 mm) and eventually reaching asystole.

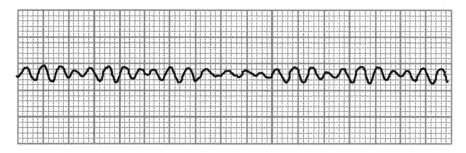

Figure 1.8. ECG: Ventricular Fibrillation (V-fib)

MANAGEMENT

- priority intervention for V-tach: check for pulse
  - □ pulseless V-tach: follow ACLS protocols
  - □ V-tach with a pulse, patient stable: administer amiodarone
  - □ V-tach with a pulse, patient unstable: synchronized cardioversion
- for V-fib: follow ACLS protocols
  - □ immediately initiate high-quality CPR at 100 – 120 compressions per minute
  - □ defibrillation ASAP, before administration of any drugs
  - □ defibrillation doses: 200 J → 300 J → 360 J (biphasic)
  - □ ≥ 2 defibrillation attempts should be made for patients in V-fib before giving any medications
  - □ first line: epinephrine 1 mg every 3 – 5 minutes
  - □ shock-refractory V-fib: amiodarone (300 mg as first dose and 150 mg for second dose)

QUICK REVIEW QUESTION

6. The nurse is participating in a cardiac resuscitation attempt of a patient found in V-fib. A total of 2 defibrillation attempts have been made, and 1 dose of epinephrine has been given 2 minutes earlier. What priority action should the nurse take next?

Pulseless Electrical Activity (PEA)/Asystole ★

PATHOPHYSIOLOGY

PULSELESS ELECTRICAL ACTIVITY (PEA) is an organized rhythm in which the heart does not contract with enough force to create a pulse. ASYSTOLE, also called a "flat line," occurs when there is no electrical or mechanical activity within the heart (Figure 1.9). Both PEA and asystole are nonshockable rhythms with a poor survival rate.

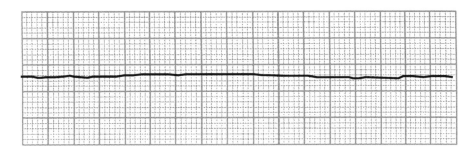

Figure 1.9. ECG: Asystole

MANAGEMENT

- immediate high-quality CPR
- epinephrine 1 mg every 3 – 5 minutes until circulation returns or a shockable rhythm emerges

- immediate attempts to determine and treat underlying cause, particularly H's and T's (common causes of PEA and asystole):
  - ☐ hypovolemia
  - ☐ hypoxia
  - ☐ hydrogen ion (acidosis)
  - ☐ hyperkalemia/hypokalemia
  - ☐ hypothermia
  - ☐ toxins
  - ☐ tamponade
  - ☐ tension pneumothorax
  - ☐ thrombosis (coronary or pulmonary)

QUICK REVIEW QUESTION

7. A patient is found in bed and is unresponsive to commands. The person appears cyanotic, and the nurse determines there is no pulse and no breathing present. What should the nurse do first?

Atrioventricular Blocks

PATHOPHYSIOLOGY

HELPFUL HINT

If the R is far from *P*, then you have a *first degree*.

Longer, longer, longer, *drop*, this is how you know it's a *Wenckebach*.

If some Ps just don't go *through*, then you know it's a *type 2*.

If Ps and Qs don't *agree*, then you have a *third degree*.

An ATRIOVENTRICULAR (AV) BLOCK is the disruption of electrical signals between the atria and ventricles. The electrical impulse may be delayed (first-degree block), intermittent (second-degree block), or completely blocked (third-degree block).

A FIRST-DEGREE AV BLOCK occurs when the conduction between the SA and the AV nodes is slowed, creating a prolonged PR interval. A first-degree AV block is a benign finding that is usually asymptomatic, but it can progress to a second-degree or third-degree block.

The ECG in a first-degree AV block will show a prolonged PR interval of > 0.20 seconds (Figure 1.10).

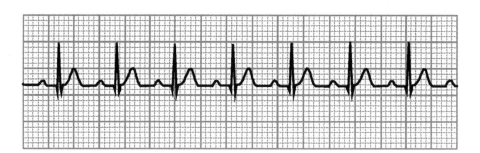

Figure 1.10. ECG: First-Degree Atrioventricular (AV) Block

A SECOND-DEGREE AV BLOCK, TYPE 1 (Wenckebach or Mobitz type 1), occurs when the PR interval progressively lengthens until the atrial impulse is completely blocked and does not produce a QRS impulse. This dysrhythmia occurs when the atrial conduction in the AV node or bundle of His is either being slowed or blocked. This type of block is cyclic; after the dropped QRS complex, the pattern will repeat itself.

The ECG in second-degree AV block, type 1, will show progressively longer PR intervals until a QRS complex completely drops (Figure 1.11).

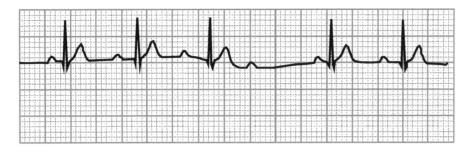

Figure 1.11. ECG: Second-Degree AV Block, Type 1

A SECOND-DEGREE **AV BLOCK, TYPE 2** (Mobitz type 2), occurs when the PR interval is constant in length but not every P wave is followed by a QRS complex. This abnormal rhythm is the result of significant conduction dysfunction within the His-Purkinje system.

The ECG in second-degree AV block, type 2, will show constant PR intervals and extra P waves, with dropped QRS complexes (Figure 1.12).

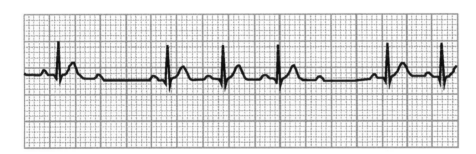

Figure 1.12. ECG: Second-Degree AV Block, Type 2

A **THIRD-DEGREE AV BLOCK**, sometimes referred to as a complete heart block, is characterized by a complete dissociation between the atria and the ventricles. There are effectively 2 pacemakers within the heart, so there is no correlation between the P waves and the QRS complexes. The most common origin of the

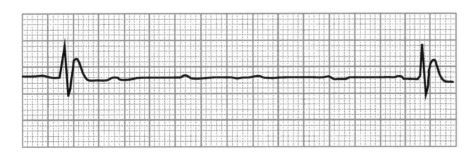

Figure 1.13. ECG: Third-Degree AV Block

block is below the bundle of His, but the block can also occur at the level of the bundle branches of the AV node.

The ECG for third-degree AV block will show regular P waves and QRS complexes that occur at different rates. There will be more P waves than QRS complexes, with P waves possibly buried within the QRS complex (Figure 1.13).

SYMPTOMS AND PHYSICAL FINDINGS

- first- and second-degree AV blocks usually asymptomatic
- may show symptoms of reduced CO (e.g., hypotension, dyspnea, chest pain)
- bradycardia

MANAGEMENT

- symptomatic patients: TCP possibly needed to manage symptoms
- implantable pacemaker if underlying cause cannot be resolved
- hypotensive patients: dopamine or epinephrine may be needed
- discontinue medications that slow electrical conduction in the heart (e.g., antidysrhythmic drugs)

QUICK REVIEW QUESTION

8. A patient begins to complain of dizziness and weakness and appears diaphoretic. The nurse notes from the telemetry monitor that the patient is in a third-degree AV block, and the blood pressure reads 71/55 mm Hg, with a heart rate of 30 bpm. What interventions does the nurse expect?

Sinus Node Dysfunction (SND)

PATHOPHYSIOLOGY

SINUS NODE DYSFUNCTION (SND), also known as sick sinus syndrome (SSS), refers to dysrhythmias caused by a dysfunction in the SA node. An individual with SND can have bouts of bradycardia or tachycardia or can alternate between the two. SND can also arise from an SA block or sinus arrest. Because of these irregular and usually unpredictable signals, most people with SND will need a permanent pacemaker.

The ECG for SND will show alternating bradycardia and tachycardia and sinus arrest (Figure 1.14).

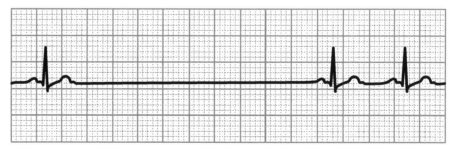

Figure 1.14. ECG: Sinus Arrest

SYMPTOMS AND PHYSICAL FINDINGS

- syncope
- fatigue
- dyspnea
- palpitations
- confusion

MANAGEMENT

- hemodynamically unstable patients: atropine and temporary pacing to correct bradycardia
- stable, asymptomatic patients: monitoring only
- symptomatic patients with recurrent episodes of bradycardia: implantable pacemaker required

QUICK REVIEW QUESTION

9. A patient with recurring episodes of bradycardia due to SND tells the nurse that they do not want to have surgery for a pacemaker, since they currently have no symptoms. What is the nurse's best response?

HELPFUL HINT
Use non-dihydropyridine calcium channel blockers, beta blockers, and antidysrhythmic drugs with caution because they may worsen SA node dysfunction.

Bundle Branch Block (BBB)

PATHOPHYSIOLOGY

RIGHT BUNDLE BRANCH BLOCK (**RBBB**) and LEFT BUNDLE BRANCH BLOCK (**LBBB**) are interruptions in conduction through a bundle branch. Bundle branch blocks (BBB) usually occur secondary to underlying cardiac conditions, including MI, hypertension, and cardiomyopathies. LBBB in particular is associated with progressive underlying structural heart disease and is associated with poor outcomes post-MI. However, both RBBB and LBBB may occur in the absence of heart disease.

Ischemic heart disease is the most common cause of both RBBB and LBBB. LBBB can also arise from other heart diseases, hyperkalemia, or digoxin toxicity. Other causes of RBBB include cor pulmonale, pulmonary edema, and myocarditis.

If the patient with a BBB is asymptomatic, no treatment is necessary. Patients with syncopal episodes may need to have a pacemaker inserted.

DID YOU KNOW?
LBBB may mask the characteristic signs of MI on an ECG.

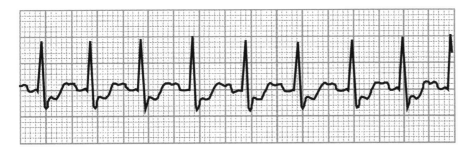

Figure 1.15. ECG: Bundle Branch Blocks (BBB)

10. A patient with HF develops a new-onset LBBB. What medication would be important to consider as a possible cause of the LBBB?

Congenital Conduction Defects

- **WOLFF-PARKINSON-WHITE SYNDROME**, caused by an early excitation of an extranodal accessary pathway, results in tachycardia.
  - asymptomatic, or presents as sudden A-fib or paroxysmal tachycardia (HR > 150)
  - ECG: short PR interval (< 0.12 seconds) with slurred QRS upstroke and wide QRS (> 0.12 seconds)
  - treatment: synchronized cardioversion; unstable patients may require catheter ablation
  - contraindications: adenosine, digoxin, amiodarone, beta blockers, calcium channel blockers

- **LONG QT SYNDROME** is a cardiac electrical disturbance that causes a prolonged ventricular repolarization (seen as a QT interval > 0.44 seconds on ECG).
  - asymptomatic, or presents with dysrhythmias (especially torsades de pointes), syncope, seizure, or sudden cardiac death
  - management: beta blockers and placement of an ICD
  - contraindications: medications likely to prolong the QT interval

- **BRUGADA SYNDROME** is a genetically inherited cardiac electrical pathway syndrome that is linked to 4 – 12% of all sudden cardiac deaths.
  - characteristic ECG findings with sudden cardiac arrest, ventricular tachydysrhythmias, or syncopal episodes to diagnose
  - ECG: pseudo-RBBB and persistent ST-segment elevation
  - ECG abnormalities may be unmasked by sodium channel blockers
  - treat with medication (quinidine or flecainide) or ICD placement
  - contraindications: medications likely to prolong the QT interval

HELPFUL HINT

Caution should be exercised when administering antipsychotics, antidepressants, and anticonvulsants if the QT is > 0.45 seconds.

11. A combative patient with schizophrenia develops torsades de pointes in the ICU. What medications may have caused this dysrhythmia?

INFECTIVE ENDOCARDITIS

PATHOPHYSIOLOGY

INFECTIVE ENDOCARDITIS occurs when an infection causes inflammation of the endocardium. The inflammation impairs valve function and may also disrupt the electrical conduction system. Infective endocarditis can occur secondary to surgical valve replacement; these cases have high a mortality rate.

DIAGNOSIS

- general signs and symptoms of infection (e.g., fever, chills, anorexia)
- petechiae
- splinter hemorrhages under fingernails
- Janeway lesions, Osler nodes, or Roth spots
- arthralgias
- dyspnea
- ECG may show dysrhythmias (A-fib or AV block most common)
- echocardiogram to assess valves
- WBC and blood cultures indicate infection

MANAGEMENT

- aggressive treatment with IV antimicrobials
- pharmacologic management of symptoms: antipyretics, diuretics, or dysrhythmics
- surgical repair of valves if necessary

QUICK REVIEW QUESTION

12. A patient is admitted with signs of infective endocarditis. What priority interventions should the nurse expect to perform?

HEART FAILURE (HF) ★

PATHOPHYSIOLOGY

HEART FAILURE (HF) occurs when either one or both of the ventricles in the heart cannot efficiently pump blood, resulting in decreased CO. The condition is typically due to another disease or illness, most commonly CAD. **ACUTE DECOMPENSATED HEART FAILURE** is the sudden onset or worsening of HF symptoms. The American Heart Association classifies HF into four stages:

- **STAGE A**: high risk of developing heart failure
- **STAGE B**: diagnosis of left systolic ventricular failure with no symptoms
- **STAGE C**: diagnosis of heart failure, with symptoms
- **STAGE D**: advanced symptoms that have not improved with treatment

HF is classified according to the left ventricular ejection fraction. Impairment of systolic function results in **HEART FAILURE WITH REDUCED EJECTION FRACTION (HFrEF, OR SYSTOLIC HF)**, classified as an ejection fraction of < 50%. **HEART FAILURE WITH PRESERVED EJECTION FRACTION (HFpEF, OR DIASTOLIC HF)** is characterized by an ejection fraction of > 50% and diastolic dysfunction.

Table 1.2. Systolic Versus Diastolic Heart Failure

SYSTOLIC HF (HFREF)	DIASTOLIC HF (HFPEF)
• reduced ejection fraction (< 50%)	• normal ejection fraction
• dilated left ventricle	• no enlargement of heart
• S3 heart sound	• S4 heart sound
• hypotension	• hypertension

HF can also be categorized as left-sided or right-sided, depending on which ventricle is affected. LEFT-SIDED HF is usually caused by cardiac disorders (e.g., MI, cardiomyopathy) and produces symptoms related to pulmonary function. RIGHT-SIDED HF is caused by right ventricle infarction or pulmonary conditions (e.g., PE, COPD) and produces symptoms related to systemic circulation. Unmanaged left-sided HF can lead to right-sided HF.

DIAGNOSIS

- BNP > 100 pg/mL
- echocardiogram and chest X-ray to assess heart function

Table 1.3. Symptoms and Physical Findings of Right- and Left-Sided Heart Failure (HF)

LEFT-SIDED HF	RIGHT-SIDED HF
• increased LVEDP and left atrial pressures	• increased right ventricular end-diastolic pressure (RVEDP) and right atrial pressures
• increased PAP	• increased CVP
• dyspnea or orthopnea	• increased PAP
• pulmonary edema	• dependent edema (usually in lower legs); ascites
• tachycardia	• JVD
• bibasilar crackles	• hepatomegaly
• cough, frothy sputum, hemoptysis	• right-sided S3 sound
• left-sided S3 sound	• weight gain
• diaphoresis	• nausea, vomiting, abdominal pain
• pulsus alternans	• nocturia
• oliguria	

MANAGEMENT

- patient needs for pharmacological and surgical interventions vary, depending on the type and degree of HF
- improve CO and CI
- medications
  - inotropics
  - vasodilators
  - ACE inhibitors, ARBs
  - digoxin

☐ diuretics

☐ beta blockers (decreases risk of sudden cardiac death)

■ other interventions: ICD, a permanent pacemaker, an IABP, a ventricular assist device (VAD), or a transplant

QUICK REVIEW QUESTION

13. A patient presents with sudden onset dyspnea, JVD, and peripheral edema. What laboratory test would confirm a diagnosis of acute decompensated heart failure?

HYPERTENSION

PATHOPHYSIOLOGY

HYPERTENSION is blood pressure > 120/80 mm Hg. Because blood pressure readings can vary, at least 2 readings on separate days must be taken to diagnose hypertension. PRIMARY (ESSENTIAL) HYPERTENSION occurs with no known cause. Primary hypertension is highly correlated with lifestyle factors, including smoking, inactivity, obesity, high alcohol intake, and a high-sodium diet. SECONDARY HYPERTENSION has a known primary cause such as medication or an endocrine disorder. Persistent hypertension can cause organ damage and is a risk factor for other cardiac disease processes.

Table 1.4. Assessing for Hypertension

CATEGORY	DESCRIPTION
Elevated blood pressure	systolic BP 120 – 129 mm Hg
	diastolic BP < 80 mm Hg
Stage 1 hypertension	systolic BP 130 – 139 mm Hg
	diastolic BP 80 – 90 mm Hg
Stage 2 hypertension	systolic BP ≥ 140 mm Hg
	diastolic BP ≥ 90 mm Hg
Hypertensive urgency	systolic BP > 180/110 mm Hg without evidence of organ dysfunction
Hypertensive crisis	systolic BP > 180 mm Hg and/or a diastolic BP > 120 mm Hg, accompanied by evidence of impending or progressive organ dysfunction

MANAGEMENT

■ initial management of chronic hypertension: lifestyle changes

☐ decreased salt intake

☐ DASH diet (high in fruits, vegetables, and lean meats; low in sugar and red meat)

☐ increased exercise

☐ weight loss

☐ reduced caffeine intake

- first-line medications: ACE inhibitors, ARBs, calcium channel blockers, and thiazide diuretics

Quick Review Question

14. A patient has an initial blood pressure reading of 160/95 mm Hg and expresses concern about being diagnosed with hypertension and needing to be on lifelong hypertensive medications. What actions should the nurse take?

PERICARDITIS

Pathophysiology

Pericarditis is the inflammation of the PERICARDIUM, the lining that surrounds the heart. When inflammation occurs, fluid can accumulate, resulting in PERICARDIAL EFFUSION. When the effusion is large enough to impair the ability of the heart to pump blood sufficiently, the condition is called PERICARDIAL TAMPONADE.

Diagnosis

- chest pain
  - □ sudden and severe
  - □ increases with movement, lying flat, and inspiration
  - □ decreases by sitting up or learning forward
  - □ radiates to neck
- pericardial friction rub
- tachycardia (usually the earliest sign)
- tachypnea or dyspnea
- fever, chills, and cough
- pericardial tamponade
  - □ Beck's triad (hypotension, JVD, muffled heart tones)
  - □ pulsus paradoxus
  - □ Kussmaul's sign
- ECG
  - □ ST elevation possible, usually in all leads except aVR and V1
  - □ tall, peaked T waves
- chest X-ray showing "water bottle" silhouette in pericardial effusion
- echocardiogram may show pericardial effusion, thickening, or calcifications

Management

- manage symptoms
  - □ pain not relieved by nitroglycerin or rest
  - □ NSAID (e.g., ibuprofen or indomethacin [Indocin])

- □ place patient in comfortable position (e.g., leaning over a bedside table)
- □ bed rest
- □ oxygen
- treat underlying conditions (e.g., antibiotics, steroids, or corticosteroids)
- pericardiocentesis or pericardial window if effusion needs to be drained
- complications: dysrhythmias, cardiac tamponade, heart failure

QUICK REVIEW QUESTION

15. A patient with acute pericarditis complains of sudden chest pain, and a pericardial friction rub can be heard on auscultation. What interventions should the nurse expect to perform to treat this patient?

ARTERIAL AND VENOUS DISEASE

Chronic Venous Insufficiency (CVI)

PATHOPHYSIOLOGY

CHRONIC VENOUS INSUFFICIENCY (CVI) occurs when the veins within the legs do not move blood effectively, because of inadequate muscle pump function, damaged venous valves, or thrombosis. Blood then pools within the veins, and blood flow to the heart is diminished. Risk factors for CVI include immobility, prolonged sitting, obesity, and pregnancy.

DIAGNOSIS

- distended vessels
- varicose veins
- lower extremity edema
- pain that increases with movement
- a feeling of tightness or stretching of the legs
- itching feeling in lower extremities
- skin discoloration
- leg muscle cramps or spasms
- venous ulcers
- venous duplex ultrasound to assess blood flow

MANAGEMENT

- most patients managed without medication or invasive procedures
    - □ elevation of legs to promote blood flow back to the heart
    - □ compression stockings to apply pressure to legs and keep blood flowing
    - □ exercise to increase circulation
    - □ higher-fiber diet to help control CVI

☐   reduced-sodium diet to prevent excess fluid accumulation

■   surgical or endovascular procedures (vein ablation or venous bypass) for patients who do not respond to noninvasive management

QUICK REVIEW QUESTION

16. The nurse is caring for a patient with CVI. What type of diet should the nurse teach the patient to follow?

Deep Vein Thrombosis (DVT)

PATHOPHYSIOLOGY

A DEEP VEIN THROMBOSIS (**DVT**) is the most common form of acute venous occlusion and occurs when a thrombus forms within a deep vein. DVT is most common in the lower extremities. Risk factors for acute venous occlusion include the following:

■   Virchow's triad:

☐   hypercoagulability (e.g., due to estrogen or contraceptive use or malignancy)

☐   venous stasis (bed rest or any other activity that results in decreased physical movement)

☐   endothelial damage (damage to the vessel wall from trauma, drug use, inflammatory processes, or other causes)

■   pregnancy, hormone replacement therapy, or oral contraceptives

■   recent surgery

DIAGNOSIS

■   pain localized to a specific area (usually the foot, ankle, or calf or behind the knee)

■   unilateral edema, erythema, and warmth

■   positive Homans sign

■   elevated D-dimer

■   venous duplex ultrasonography to diagnose

MANAGEMENT

■   first line: anticoagulants

■   second line: thrombolytics

■   surgical or endovascular thrombectomy may be required

■   inferior vena cava filter may be placed to avoid a pulmonary embolism (PE) in patients who cannot tolerate anticoagulants

QUICK REVIEW QUESTION

17. A patient diagnosed with a DVT complains of dyspnea. The nurse knows the priority invention for this patient is what?

Peripheral Vascular Insufficiency

PATHOPHYSIOLOGY

Atherosclerosis that occurs in peripheral arteries leads to PERIPHERAL VASCULAR INSUFFICIENCY (also called peripheral arterial disease [PAD]). ACUTE PERIPHERAL VASCULAR INSUFFICIENCY (also ACUTE ARTERIAL OCCLUSION) occurs when a thrombus or an embolus occludes a peripheral artery and causes ischemia and possibly the loss of a limb. This condition is a medical emergency requiring prompt treatment to prevent tissue necrosis.

DIAGNOSIS

- the 6 Ps (hallmark signs) of an arterial occlusion:
  - ☐ pain (intermittent claudication)
  - ☐ pallor
  - ☐ pulselessness
  - ☐ paresthesia
  - ☐ paralysis
  - ☐ poikilothermia
- petechiae (visible with microemboli)
- ABPI < 0.30 (indicating poor outcome of limb survivability)
- duplex ultrasonography, CT angiography, or catheter-based arteriography to diagnosis
- elevated D-dimer

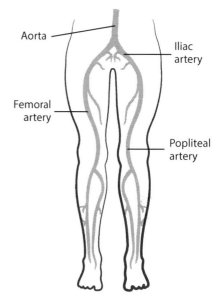

Figure 1.16. Common Locations of Acute Arterial Occlusion

MANAGEMENT

- pharmacological management: thrombolytics, anticoagulants (e.g., heparin), and antiplatelet agents
- other interventions: embolectomy, catheter-directed thrombolysis, or bypass surgery
- nursing considerations for arterial occlusion:
  - ☐ frequent pulse and neurovascular checks to monitor for worsening of condition or other changes
  - ☐ do not elevate extremity or apply heat
  - ☐ thrombolytic therapy, typically for 4 – 24 hours; reevaluation via angiogram; monitoring for symptoms and physical findings of bleeding

QUICK REVIEW QUESTION

18. Catheter-directed thrombolysis is performed on a patient with an acute arterial occlusion in the lower right leg. What nursing interventions are the most important?

CARDIAC TRAUMA

PATHOPHYSIOLOGY

CARDIAC TRAUMA can occur when an outside force causes injury to the heart. Cardiac trauma can cause rupture of heart chambers, dysrhythmias, damage to the heart valves, or cardiac arrest. Blunt cardiac trauma and penetrating cardiac trauma can both be fatal.

BLUNT CARDIAC TRAUMA occurs when an object forcefully strikes the chest. Because the atria and right ventricle are anteriorly positioned, they are typically the most affected. Blunt trauma to the heart causes a decrease in the right ventricle contractility and ejection fraction. In blunt cardiac trauma, the heart is compressed between the sternum and the spine. Sudden cardiac death can also occur from blunt trauma.

PENETRATING CARDIAC TRAUMA involves the puncture of the heart by a sharp object or by a broken rib. The most frequently affected area is the right ventricle. The penetration causes blood to leak into the pericardial space or mediastinum; the leakage can result in cardiac tamponade. Fluid or blood loss from penetrating injuries can also result in shock.

TREATMENT AND MANAGEMENT

- medications for blunt trauma: inotropes (e.g., dobutamine), anti-inflammatories, opioids
- penetrating objects should be stabilized and the patient prepped for surgery
- monitor for and treat complications:
    □ dysrhythmias
    □ cardiac tamponade
    □ valve or ventricular rupture
    □ heart failure
    □ cardiogenic shock
    □ hemothorax
    □ pneumothorax

QUICK REVIEW QUESTION

19. A patient arrives at the ED with a knife impaled in the chest. The patient is awake and alert but anxious and appears pale. What priority interventions should the nurse perform?

SHOCK (CARDIOGENIC)

PATHOPHYSIOLOGY

CARDIOGENIC SHOCK, a cyclical decline in cardiac function, results in decreased cardiac output (CO) in the presence of adequate fluid volume. A lack of coronary perfusion causes or escalates ischemia/infarction by decreasing the ability of the heart to pump effectively. The heart rate increases in an attempt to meet myocardial oxygen demands. However, the reduced pumping ability of the heart reduces CO and the cardiac index (CI), and demands for coronary or tissue perfusion are not met. Left ventricular end-diastolic pressure (LVEDP) increases, which leads to stress in the left ventricle and an increase in afterload. This distress results in lactic acidosis. Cardiogenic shock is most commonly seen after an MI but can be associated with trauma, infection, or metabolic disease.

DIAGNOSIS

- tachycardia and sustained hypotension (SBP < 90 mm Hg)
- oliguria (< 30 mL/ hr or < 0.5 mL/kg/hour output)
- crackles
- tachypnea and dyspnea
- pallor and cool, clammy skin
- JVD
- altered LOC
- S3 heart sound possible
- CI < 2.2 L/min/m^2
- PAOP > 15 mm Hg
- elevated SVR, CVP
- decreased SvO$_2$, MAP
- elevated lactate
- ABG shows metabolic acidosis and hypoxia

TREATMENT AND MANAGEMENT

- main treatment goal: to identify and treat underlying cause and to reduce cardiac workload and improve myocardial contractility
- immediate IV fluids
- medications
  - □ dobutamine or norepinephrine (to increase contractility and CO)
  - □ antiplatelet drugs (e.g., aspirin or clopidogrel)
  - □ thrombolytic drugs (e.g., alteplase [Activase] or reteplase)
  - □ morphine
  - □ nitroprusside (Nipride)
- other interventions
  - □ IABP to reduce afterload and increase coronary perfusion
  - □ cardiac catheterization to improve myocardial perfusion and increase contractility
  - □ left ventricular assist device
- monitor patient for cardiac dysrhythmias

20. A patient presents with tachycardia, pallor, JVD, and crackles after emergent PCI for anterior MI. What hemodynamic findings for this patient would indicate cardiogenic shock?

ANSWER KEY

1. The main priority for this patient is obtaining a 12-lead ECG to rule out a STEMI. Additional priorities include obtaining labs, specifically a troponin and electrolyte panel; monitoring the patient's vital signs; applying oxygen if the person is hypoxic; and placing the patient on telemetry to continuously monitor cardiac rhythm.

2. Since the patient describes the pain as tearing, the nurse should take the blood pressure in the other arm. A difference of ≥ 20 mm Hg can be a strong indicator that the patient is experiencing an aortic rupture or dissection.

3. This patient is hemodynamically unstable because of bradycardia. The nurse should prepare to push IV atropine.

4. If the patient in SVT does not respond to vagal maneuvers, the patient will likely be administered 6 mg of adenosine to terminate the dysrhythmia.

5. The nurse should expect a hemodynamically stable patient with A-fib to receive calcium channel blockers, beta blockers, or cardiac glycosides to decrease the heart rate.

6. After 2 defibrillation attempts and the first dose of epinephrine has been given, the nurse should prepare the first dose of amiodarone (300 mg) to be given next.

7. The nurse should activate the code team and begin high-quality compressions immediately. (CPR should not be delayed to administer epinephrine.)

8. The nurse should prepare the patient for TCP. Dopamine and epinephrine may be appropriate medications to administer for a third-degree block as they will increase the overall heart rate.

9. The nurse should explain that the absence of symptoms does not mean that underlying conditions are gone. Without the pacemaker, the patient risks developing additional dysrhythmias or could go into sudden cardiac arrest without warning.

10. Digoxin, often administered for treatment of HF, has a narrow therapeutic index. Digoxin toxicity may manifest itself as an LBBB. Labs would need to be drawn to assess for digoxin toxicity.

11. There is a strong association between antipsychotic medication use and torsades de pointes in patients with prolonged QT. The patient may have been administered haloperidol, which is one of the most commonly used medications in the ICU associated with torsades de pointes.

12. The nurse should expect orders to get an ECG and draw labs to monitor the patient's WBC count, sedimentation rate, and C-reactive protein and to collect at least 2 sets of blood cultures. The nurse should also expect to administer antibiotics after the blood cultures have been drawn.

13. A BNP lab value of > 100 pg/mL indicates HF.

14. The nurse should make sure that the correct cuff size is being used and should check the blood pressure a second time, preferably on the opposite arm unless contraindicated. The nurse can also inform the patient that a diagnosis

of hypertension must be made after 2 separate elevated blood pressures are confirmed on 2 separate days.

15. The nurse should obtain a 12-lead ECG and then have the patient sit up and lean forward, a position that can help reduce the pain. The nurse can also administer an NSAID such as ibuprofen or indomethacin to assist with pain control and reduce inflammation.

16. The patient with CVI should follow a low-sodium, high-fiber diet to reduce fluid buildup.

17. Patients with DVT and dyspnea should immediately have a CT scan ordered to rule out a PE. A PE is an emergent condition that needs immediate treatment.

18. The nurse should ensure strict bedrest and make sure that the affected extremity is kept straight. The nurse should also assess the site frequently and notify the physician for bleeding, coldness, increased pain, or decreased pulse. NPO status should be initiated 8 hours before reevaluation.

19. Any patient with a penetrating object injury should have the nurse ensure that the object is stabilized but not removed. Bleeding should be controlled, and 2 large-bore IVs should be placed for the administration of IV fluids and blood if needed. The patient should be prepped for surgery to have the object removed and to be assessed for underlying damage to organs and surrounding areas.

20. Cardiogenic shock is characterized by signs and symptoms of hypoperfusion combined with a systolic BP of < 90 mm Hg, a CI of < 2.2 L/min/m^2, and a normal or elevated PAOP (> 15 mm Hg).

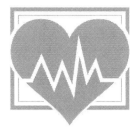

2

RESPIRATORY EMERGENCIES

BCEN CONTENT OUTLINE

  A. Aspiration

✷ **B. ASTHMA**

✷ **C. CHRONIC OBSTRUCTIVE PULMONARY DISEASE (COPD)**

✷ **D. INFECTIONS**

  E. Inhalation injuries

  F. Obstruction

  G. Pleural effusion

  H. Pneumothorax

  I. Pulmonary edema, noncardiac

✷ **J. PULMONARY EMBOLUS**

  K. Respiratory distress syndrome

  L. Trauma

ASPIRATION

PATHOPHYSIOLOGY

PULMONARY ASPIRATION is the entry of foreign bodies, or material from the mouth or gastrointestinal tract, into the upper and/or lower respiratory tract. Risk factors for aspiration include recent surgery, intoxication, sedation, or altered LOC.

DIAGNOSIS

- coughing or choking
- dyspnea

- lung sounds may be decreased in the lobe in which the aspiration has settled
- crackles may be heard if fluid was aspirated
- chest X-ray showing infiltrates after the aspiration
- WBC and blood cultures may show infection

TREATMENT AND MANAGEMENT

- manage airway
- oxygen and antibiotics as needed

QUICK REVIEW QUESTION

1. A patient presents to the ED with pleuritic chest pain, difficulty breathing, fevers, chills, and an altered LOC. The patient's friend alerts the triage nurse that 3 days ago, the patient was found in a pool of vomit after an overdose. What should the nurse anticipate for this patient?

ASTHMA

ASTHMA, an obstructive disease of the lungs, is characterized by long-term inflammation and constriction of the bronchial airways. Patients with asthma often experience exacerbations triggered by lung irritants, exercise, stress, or allergies.

STATUS ASTHMATICUS is a severe condition in which the patient is experiencing intractable asthma exacerbations with limited pauses or no pause between the exacerbations. The symptoms are unresponsive to initial treatment and can ultimately lead to acute respiratory failure. Status asthmaticus can develop over hours or days.

DIAGNOSIS

- tachypnea and severe dyspnea
- wheezing
  - □ expiratory wheeze (early stage)
  - □ inspiratory and expiratory wheeze (late stage)
- increased use of accessory respiratory muscles
- decreased breath sounds in all lung fields (ominous sign, as patient is not moving enough air)
- tachycardia and hypertension
- pulsus paradoxus > 20 mm Hg
- peak expiratory flow rate (PEFR) showing 20% drop from baseline best effort
- ABG:
  - □ initial: respiratory alkalosis with hypoxemia

□ worsening: respiratory acidosis with hypercapnia

■ CXR to rule out other underlying diseases (e.g., pneumonia, pneumothorax)

TREATMENT AND MANAGEMENT

■ medication
 □ inhaled bronchodilators (beta 2 agonists): albuterol
 □ anticholinergics (synergistic effect with beta 2 agonists): ipratropium inhalation (Atrovent)
 □ corticosteroids: methylprednisolone (IV) or prednisone (PO)

■ oxygen: high-flow treatment to keep SpO_2 > 92 %, or heliox to decrease airway resistance

■ mechanical ventilation for refractory status asthmaticus

QUICK REVIEW QUESTION

2. A patient arrives via EMS for acute asthma exacerbation. Upon arrival, the patient is breathing rapidly, is unable to speak in full sentences, and appears anxious. What is the first action the nurse should take in the care of this patient?

CHRONIC OBSTRUCTIVE PULMONARY DISEASE (COPD)

★

CHRONIC OBSTRUCTIVE PULMONARY DISEASE (**COPD**) is characterized by a breakdown in alveolar tissue (emphysema), chronic productive cough (chronic bronchitis), and long-term obstruction of the airways; the condition worsens

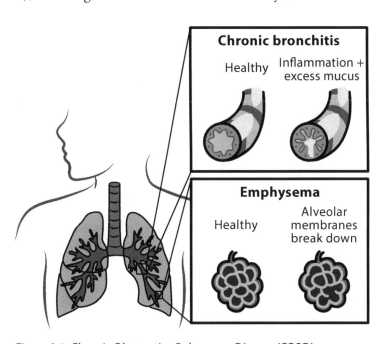

Figure 2.1. Chronic Obstructive Pulmonary Disease (COPD)

over time. COPD is characterized by low expiratory flow rates. Acute exacerbations of COPD are characterized by increased sputum production and hypoxia or hypercapnia, which may require emergent treatment.

DIAGNOSIS

- chronic, productive cough
- dyspnea and wheezing
- prolonged expiration
- barrel chest (late sign)

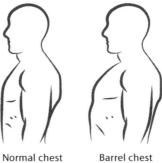

Normal chest   Barrel chest

Figure 2.2. Barrel Chest

TREATMENT AND MANAGEMENT

HELPFUL HINT

In COPD, inflammation is mainly caused by neutrophils. In asthma, inflammation is caused by eosinophils and activated T cells. Corticosteroids are highly effective against eosinophilic inflammation but mostly ineffective against neutrophilic inflammation.

- first-line management
  - □ bronchodilators (*not* inhaled corticosteroids) such as short-acting beta-agonists (e.g., albuterol)
  - □ anticholinergics with cautious use of oxygen (titrated to SaO_2 88 – 92% or PaO_2 of 60 mm Hg)
- monitor for hypercapnia when administering oxygen
- chest physiotherapy and comfortable positioning
- teach smoking cessation at discharge

QUICK REVIEW QUESTION

3. A 50-year-old patient has been newly diagnosed with COPD and is anxious about the diagnosis. The patient wants to know if there is a cure for COPD. How should the nurse respond?

★ INFECTIONS

- **PNEUMONIA** is a lower respiratory tract infection that can be caused by bacteria, fungi, protozoa, or parasites. The infection causes inflammation in the alveoli and can cause them to fill with fluid.
  - □ Diagnosis and treatment of community-acquired pneumonia (CAP), hospital-acquired pneumonia (HAP), and aspiration pneumonia are similar.

□ Signs and symptoms include cough, dyspnea, hemoptysis, pleuritic chest pain, and fever. Abnormalities in affected lung/lobe include decreased lung sounds, inspiratory crackles, and dull percussion.

□ Chest X-ray will show infiltrates; WBC and blood cultures will show infection.

□ Management is antibiotics and oxygen as needed.

■ **CROUP** is an upper airway obstruction caused by subglottic inflammation that results from viral illness (although rarely it can be caused by bacterial infection). The inflammation results in edema in the trachea and adjacent structures. Additionally, thick, tenacious mucus further obstructs the airway.

□ Croup is associated with a barking cough and characteristic high-pitched stridor.

□ Management may include oxygen, cool mist therapy, corticosteroids, dexamethasone, and nebulized racemic epinephrine.

■ **BRONCHITIS** is inflammation of the bronchi. Most cases (> 90%) are caused by a viral infection, but bronchitis can also result from bacterial infection or environmental irritants.

□ Signs and symptoms may include nonproductive cough that evolves into a productive cough, sore throat, and congestion.

□ Acute bronchitis will usually spontaneously resolve without intervention.

□ Fluids, antitussives, analgesics, or antibiotics may be administered.

■ **BRONCHIOLITIS** is inflammation of the bronchioles, usually because of infection by RSV or human rhinovirus. The inflammation and congestion lead to a narrowing of the airway, resulting in dyspnea. Bronchiolitis is seen in children younger than 2 years and will usually spontaneously resolve.

HELPFUL HINT

In patients with unilateral lung disease (e.g., right lung pneumonia), the patient should be positioned with the "good" lung down to promote blood flow and perfusion in the healthy lung.

QUICK REVIEW QUESTION

4. The mother of an 18-month-old is concerned that her child has pneumonia. She asks the nurse to describe the difference between a diagnosis of pneumonia and a diagnosis of bronchiolitis. How should the nurse respond?

INHALATION INJURIES
PATHOPHYSIOLOGY

INHALATION INJURIES fall into three categories differentiated by the mechanism of the injury:

■ Exposure to asphyxiants such as carbon monoxide (CO) can cause injuries. In the case of CO poisoning, the CO displaces the oxygen on the hemoglobin molecule, leading to hypoxia and eventual death of tissue.

- Thermal or heat inhalation injuries can be caused by steam, heat from explosions, or the consumption of very hot liquids. The resulting edema and blistering of the airway mucosa lead to airway obstruction.
- Smoke exposure from fire or toxic gases causes damage to pulmonary tissue and causes mucosal edema and the destruction of epithelia cilia. Pulmonary edema is a late development, one to two days after the injury.

DIAGNOSIS

- depends on what irritant the patient is exposed to
- mucosal and pulmonary edema possible up to 48 hours after exposure
- general s/s of respiratory distress (e.g., dyspnea, wheezing, etc.)

TREATMENT AND MANAGEMENT

- manage airway
- oxygen as needed
- administer antidote if available
- vigorous pulmonary hygiene with patient (including suctioning of airways, blow bottles, and nasotracheal suction)

QUICK REVIEW QUESTION

5. EMS arrives with a patient who was rescued from a home fire. The patient is unconscious, but the airway is currently clear and intact. Assessment of the airway reveals black soot at the opening of the mouth and at the nares. What is the next nursing consideration for this patient?

OBSTRUCTION

PATHOPHYSIOLOGY

AIRWAY OBSTRUCTION, or blockage of the upper airway, can be caused by a foreign body (e.g., teeth, food, marbles), the tongue, vomit, blood, or other secretions. Possible causes of airway obstruction include traumatic injuries to the face, edema in the airway, peritonsillar abscess, and burns to the airway. Small children may also place foreign bodies in their mouths or obstruct their airway with food.

DIAGNOSIS

- visually observed obstruction in airway
- dyspnea or gasping for air
- stridor
- excessive drooling in infants
- agitation or panic
- loss of consciousness, altered LOC, or respiratory arrest

- suction mouth and upper airway

- rapid intubation or cricothyrotomy where appropriate

QUICK REVIEW QUESTION

6. In what order should the nurse perform an airway assessment in a patient with a suspected foreign body obstruction?

PLEURAL EFFUSION

PATHOPHYSIOLOGY

A **PLEURAL EFFUSION** is the buildup of fluid around the lungs in the pleural space. This fluid buildup can displace lung tissue and inhibit adequate ventilation and lung expansion. There are two types of pleural effusions:

- Transudative pleural effusions occur when fluid leaks into the pleural space. They can be caused by low serum protein levels or increased systemic pressure in the vessels.

- Exudative pleural effusions are due to blockage of blood or lymph vessels, tumors, lung injury, or inflammation.

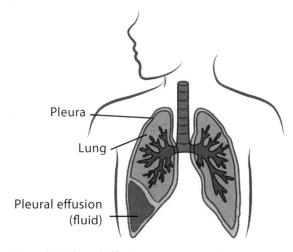

Figure 2.3. Pleural Effusion

DIAGNOSIS

- dyspnea

- dullness upon percussion of the lung area

- asymmetrical chest expansion

- decreased breath sounds on affected side

- cough (dry or productive)

- pleuritic chest pain

- chest X-ray showing white areas at the base of the lungs (unilaterally or bilaterally)
- CT scan to further diagnose the severity of the condition
- thoracentesis to determine the mechanism of effusion

TREATMENT AND MANAGEMENT

- drainage of excess pleural fluid where appropriate
- medications based underlying condition
    - diuretics (to assist with reducing effusion size)
    - antibiotics (for infection)

QUICK REVIEW QUESTION

7. A nursing student requests assistance with understanding the difference between pulmonary effusion and ARDS. What is your response?

PNEUMOTHORAX

PATHOPHYSIOLOGY

PNEUMOTHORAX is the collection of air between the chest wall and the lung (pleural space). It can occur from blunt chest-wall injury, medical injury, underlying lung tissue disease, or hereditary factors. Pneumothorax is classified according to its underlying cause:

- **PRIMARY SPONTANEOUS PNEUMOTHORAX (PSP)** occurs spontaneously in the absence of lung disease and often presents with only minor symptoms.
- **SECONDARY SPONTANEOUS PNEUMOTHORAX (SSP)** occurs in patients with an underlying lung disease and presents with more severe symptoms.
- **TRAUMATIC PNEUMOTHORAX** occurs when the chest wall is penetrated.
- **TENSION PNEUMOTHORAX**, the late progression of a pneumothorax, causes significant respiratory distress in the patient and requires immediate intervention for treatment.

DIAGNOSIS

- sudden unilateral chest pain
- dyspnea
- tachycardia
- hypoxia and cyanosis
- hypotension
- tension pneumothorax:
    - tracheal deviation away from the side of the tension
    - decreased breath sounds on the affected side
    - increased percussion note

HELPFUL HINT

Pneumothorax presents with tracheal deviation <u>toward</u> affected side. Tension pneumothorax presents with tracheal deviation <u>away from</u> unaffected side.

☐   distended neck veins

■   chest X-ray will show lung tissue separated from the chest wall

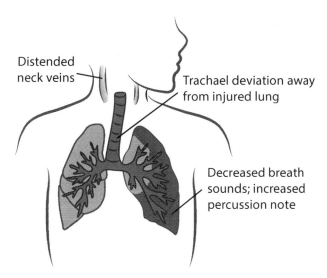

Distended
neck veins

Trachael deviation away
from injured lung

Decreased breath
sounds; increased
percussion note

Figure 2.4. Signs and Symptoms of Tension Pneumothorax

TREATMENT AND MANAGEMENT

■   pneumothorax < 15%: supplemental oxygen and monitoring

■   pneumothorax > 15%: percutaneous needle aspiration of air from pleural
    space and insertion of chest tube:

    ☐   insertion at fourth or fifth intercostal space mid-axillary line on
        affected side

    ☐   water-seal drainage system or Heimlich valve

    ☐   CXR to confirm lung re-expansion

■   emergent treatment of tension pneumothorax: immediate percutaneous
    placement of large-bore needle (insertion at second intercostal space
    mid-axillary line on affected side) and chest-tube insertion

QUICK REVIEW QUESTION

8.   A patient with blunt thoracic trauma has been diagnosed with pneumothorax
     and was alert and oriented upon arrival via EMS. On reassessment of the
     patient, the nurse finds the patient restless and anxious. The patient also
     has tachypnea and tachycardia, with visually distended neck veins. What
     intervention should the nurse anticipate?

PULMONARY EDEMA (NONCARDIAC)

PATHOPHYSIOLOGY

NONCARDIAC PULMONARY EDEMA (NPE) is when fluid collects in the alveoli
of the lungs, but the condition is not due to heart failure. This fluid inhibits
gas exchange. NPE can be caused by a wide range of injuries and underlying
disorders, including:

- CNS injury (NEUROGENIC PULMONARY EDEMA)
- removal of airway obstruction (POSTOBSTRUCTIVE PULMONARY EDEMA)
- rapid increase in altitude (HIGH-ALTITUDE PULMONARY EDEMA)
- reexpansion of the lung (REEXPANSION PULMONARY EDEMA)
- aspiration
- inhalation of toxic gases
- immersion injuries

DIAGNOSIS

- frothy pink pulmonary secretions
- dyspnea or orthopnea
- cough (dry or productive)
- chest pain
- fatigue, weakness, or dizziness
- tachypnea
- hypoxia
- crackles
- chest X-ray showing white appearance over both lung fields
- elevated plasma BNP

TREATMENT AND MANAGEMENT

- primary treatment: oxygen as needed
- secondary treatment to address underlying condition

QUICK REVIEW QUESTION

9. Which is the most effective treatment of high-altitude pulmonary edema?

PULMONARY EMBOLUS

HELPFUL HINT

PE may trigger bronchoconstriction and disrupt surfactant functioning, resulting in atelectasis (collapse of the lung).

A **PULMONARY EMBOLISM (PE)** occurs when an embolus occludes an artery of the lungs. The most common embolus is a blood clot caused by deep vein thrombosis (DVT), but tumor emboli, fat emboli, and amniotic fluid emboli can also reach the lungs. PE is an emergent condition that can result in hypoxemia, pulmonary hypertension, right ventricular failure, and decreased cardiac output.

DIAGNOSIS

- pleuritic chest pain
- dyspnea and tachypnea
- cough and/or hemoptysis
- tachycardia

- hypotension
- anxiety
- D-dimer positive (> 500 ng/mL)
- chest X-ray often normal (but collected to rule out other disease processes)
- CTPA showing evidence of PE
- spiral CT scan: a 30-second study with > 90% sensitivity/specificity
- pulmonary angiogram: definitive diagnosis but with long study time

TREATMENT AND MANAGEMENT

- IV fluid resuscitation
- IV anticoagulation (heparin) once diagnosis is confirmed
- thrombolytic drugs (fibrinolytics) for unstable patients with no contraindications
- supportive treatment for symptoms
  - O_2 therapy
  - analgesics
  - vasopressors to manage blood pressure

QUICK REVIEW QUESTION

10. A 52-year-old patient is admitted with tachycardia, tachypnea, hemoptysis, and chest pain. The patient is currently hemodynamically stable, and a diagnosis of a PE is suspected. What diagnostic study should the nurse expect to be ordered to confirm the diagnosis?

RESPIRATORY DISTRESS SYNDROME

PATHOPHYSIOLOGY

ACUTE RESPIRATORY DISTRESS SYNDROME (**ARDS**) is a sudden and progressive form of NPE in which the alveoli fill with fluid because of damage to the pulmonary endothelium. ARDS is the systemic response to a direct or indirect injury to the lungs. It is a secondary disease initiated by the inflammatory-immune system, which releases inflammatory mediators from the site of injury within 24 – 48 hours.

DIAGNOSIS

- tachypnea with increased accessory-muscle usage for work of breathing
- elevated PAP
- pulmonary artery occlusion pressure (PAOP) normal or low
- progressive hypoxemia
- lungs clear initially; fine crackles as ARDS progresses
- decreased urine output

HELPFUL HINT
ARDS is often considered a pulmonary marker of MODS, which is the leading cause of death for ARDS patients.

- tachycardia and hypotension
- CXR showing pulmonary infiltrates, ground-glass opacity, and an elevated diaphragm
- ABG findings:
  - □ decreasing P/F ratio
  - □ refractory hypoxemia
  - □ increasing hypercarbia
- lab results
  - □ lactic acidosis
  - □ elevated SGOT, ALP, bilirubin
  - □ increased PT/PTT
  - □ decreased albumin

TREATMENT AND MANAGEMENT

- simultaneous treatment of underlying cause while managing ARDS symptoms
- oxygen supplementation
- prone positioning to reduce damage to dependent areas of lungs
- intubation and mechanical ventilation likely
- careful hydration in the presence of hypovolemia

QUICK REVIEW QUESTION

11. A patient presents to the emergency department with hypotension, fever, chills, and an altered LOC. The nurse identifies that the patient is experiencing sepsis. What signs and symptoms should the nurse look for to determine if the patient has ARDS?

RESPIRATORY TRAUMA

PATHOPHYSIOLOGY

Chest trauma, whether from blunt injury; sharp, invasive penetration; or thoracic surgical procedures, creates a wide range of pulmonary complications.

TREATMENT AND MANAGEMENT

- pain management as needed
- small contusions: heal in 3 – 5 days, often without treatment
- severe contusions: may require mechanical ventilation, fluid management (to avoid overload), and infection prevention
- hemothorax: chest-tube insertion or thoracotomy (if bleeding cannot be managed)
- tracheal perforation: maintain airway, and prepare patient for surgical repair

Table 2.1. Thoracic Injuries

PATHOPHYSIOLOGY	CLINICAL PRESENTATION
PULMONARY CONTUSION Bruising of the parenchyma of the lung. Capillary rupture causes blood and other fluid to leak into lung tissue, causes localized edema, and may result in hypoxia from diminished gas exchange. Fluid accumulation in alveoli and decreased pulmonary secretion clearance put patients at risk for ARDS and pneumonia.	• signs and symptoms may be delayed 24 – 72 hours until edema develops • hemoptysis (pink, frothy sputum) • crackles • tachypnea and tachycardia • hypoxia • chest wall bruising • pain • decreased $PaCO_2$ • decreased P/F ratio
RIB FRACTURES Commonly caused by traumatic crushing injury to chest or cancer; leads to altered ventilation and perfusion status from acute. Most common fractures are ribs 4 – 8. Ribs 9 – 12 may cause splenic rupture and tears to the diaphragm and liver.	• pain with breathing • shallow breaths • splinting
HEMOTHORAX Blood in the pleural space, usually resulting from blunt or penetrating trauma to the chest wall. Damage to the lung parenchyma and great vessels causes alveoli collapse. May also present with pneumothorax (pneumohemothorax).	• symptomatic with blood volume > 400 mL • absence of breath sounds on affected side • tracheal deviation toward unaffected side • dullness to percussion • tachypnea • hypovolemia • shock
TRACHEAL RUPTURE (or PERFORATION) Occurs when there is injury to the structure of the trachea. The perforation can be caused by forceful or poor intubation efforts or by traumatic injury to the trachea such as in crush injuries or hanging injuries.	• hemoptysis • dyspnea • diffuse subcutaneous emphysema

QUICK REVIEW QUESTION

12. A 46-year-old patient with A-fib who is on anticoagulant medication suffered a fall from a small step stool in the kitchen. He had no head injury or loss of consciousness. 24 hours later, the patient is admitted with the following symptoms: pink frothy sputum, crackles in the lung fields, tachypnea, tachycardia, and pain. Ecchymosis is evident over ribs 4 – 8. ABG shows hypoxia. CXR has ruled out rib fractures but is not remarkable. The patient is sent for a chest CT scan. What diagnosis would the CCRN expect, and why was a chest CT scan ordered?

ANSWER KEY

1. The nurse should be concerned with protecting the patient's airway, but he should also prepare the patient for a chest X-ray to determine if the patient has aspirated after the vomiting. The nurse should also be prepared to suction the patient's airway in case the patient vomits again.

2. The nurse should apply oxygen via non-rebreather mask to support the patient's oxygen needs and prepare to administer nebulized albuterol and ipratropium.

3. The nurse should explain that the damage done to the lung tissue of people diagnosed with COPD is often irreversible. However, disease progression can be slowed or halted if the patient stops smoking and adheres to the prescribed regimen of medications and therapy.

4. The nurse should inform the mother that bronchiolitis does not present on X-ray with the same findings as pneumonia. If applicable, the nurse can also tell the mother that the health care team performed labs to rule out common underlying causes of pneumonia and/or to confirm the presence of the viruses that cause bronchiolitis.

5. The nurse should administer oxygen to the patient, place the patient on monitors, and alert the provider of the assessment findings. Soot at mucosal openings is a sign of possible inhalation injury and impeding edema formation in the airway, and early intubation should be considered before the airway closes and a cricothyrotomy is needed.

6. (1) Inspect the airway; (2) suction out any visible foreign bodies; and (3) reassess the patency of the airway. If the airway is still obstructed, the nurse should view directly with a laryngoscope. If all attempts fail, cricothyrotomy must be performed to open the airway.

7. Pulmonary effusion and ARDS differ in which lung structures are affected. In a pulmonary effusion, fluid collects in the pleural space that surrounds the lung and limits the ability of the lungs to expand. In ARDS, pulmonary capillary permeability is compromised, and fluid fills the alveolar sacs within the lungs. The fluid limits the ability of the lungs to exchange oxygen and carbon dioxide.

8. The nurse would suspect tension pneumothorax and should prepare to assist the provider with a needle thoracostomy to relieve the tension and to allow the lung to expand within the thorax.

9. The patient should be given oxygen therapy and should be removed to a lower altitude to address the underlying cause of the NPE.

10. Definitive diagnosis of a PE is by pulmonary angiogram. Because the patient is stable, a faster but less definitive test is unlikely to be ordered.

11. The patient with ARDS will have tachycardia, tachypnea, dyspnea, and crackles on auscultation. Measurement of the patient's vital signs will show hypoxia, and ABG will show a decreased P/F ratio. The nurse should anticipate a chest X-ray to confirm or rule out ARDS.

12. The more sensitive chest CT scan will confirm a diagnosis of pulmonary contusion.

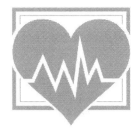

3

NEUROLOGICAL EMERGENCIES

BCEN CONTENT OUTLINE

   A. Alzheimer's disease/dementia

   B. Chronic neurological disorders (e.g., multiple sclerosis, myasthenia gravis)

   C. Guillain-Barré syndrome

★ **D. HEADACHE** (e.g., temporal arteritis, migraine)

★ **E. INCREASED INTRACRANIAL PRESSURE (ICP)**

   F. Meningitis

★ **G. SEIZURE DISORDERS**

   H. Shunt dysfunctions

   I. Spinal cord injuries, including neurogenic shock

★ **J. STROKE** (ischemic or hemorrhagic)

   K. Transient ischemic attack (TIA)

   L. Trauma

CHRONIC NEUROLOGICAL DISORDERS

- **ALZHEIMER'S DISEASE** is a cognitive deterioration caused by beta-amyloid deposits and neurofibrillary tangles in the cerebral cortex and subcortical gray matter of the brain. The most common cause for ED visits in patients with Alzheimer's is agitation or aggression.
  - ☐ Signs and Symptoms: loss of short-term memory; impaired reasoning and judgment; language dysfunction; inability to recognize faces and common objects; behavioral disturbances
  - ☐ Management: supportive treatment for symptoms; assess for the most common causes of agitation and aggression (UTI, pain, underlying

HELPFUL HINT

Antipsychotic medications, especially Haloperidol lactate (Haldol), are used cautiously in geriatric patients with dementia because they increase the risk of stroke, MI, and death.

medical condition, medications); olanzapine (Zyprexa) is the preferred medication for geriatric patients in acute crises; lorazepam (Ativan) or diphenhydramine (Benadryl) may be given

DID YOU KNOW?
Bulbar muscle weakness caused by ALS puts patients at high risk for aspiration and airway obstruction.

- **AMYOTROPHIC LATERAL SCLEROSIS (ALS)** (Lou Gehrig's disease) is a neuro-degenerative disorder that affects the neurons in the brain stem and spinal cord. Symptoms progressively worsen until respiratory failure occurs.

  - Signs and Symptoms: progressive asymmetrical weakness (can affect both upper and lower extremities); difficulty swallowing, walking, or speaking; muscle cramps

  - Management: supportive treatment for symptoms; respiratory support; high risk of aspiration

- **GUILLAIN-BARRÉ SYNDROME** is an autoimmune disorder in which the immune system attacks healthy cells within the nervous system, rapidly affecting motor function. Muscle weakness may lead to respiratory dysfunction.

  - Signs and Symptoms: neuropathy and weakness ascending from lower extremities and advancing symmetrically upward; paresthesia in extremities; unsteady gait; absent or diminished deep tendon reflexes; dyspnea; autonomic dysfunction (hypertension, bradycardia, asystole)

  - Management: analgesics; IV immunoglobulins; treatment of dysrhythmias; respiratory support

- **MULTIPLE SCLEROSIS (MS)** is a neurodegenerative disorder caused by patches of demyelination in the brain and the spinal cord. It as periods of both remission and exacerbation of symptoms with gradually growing disability.

  - Signs and Symptoms: paresthesia; weakness of at least one extremity; visual, motor, or urinary disturbance; vertigo; fatigue; mild cognitive impairment; increased deep tendon reflexes; positive Babinski sign; clonus

  - Management: corticosteroids for inflammation; baclofen (Lioresal) or tizanidine (Zanaflex) for spasticity; gabapentin (Neurontin) or tricyclic antidepressants for pain

- **MUSCULAR DYSTROPHY (MD)** is a genetic disorder in which a mutation in the recessive dystrophin gene on the X chromosome causes muscle fiber degeneration. It results in progressive proximal muscle weakness.

  - Signs and Symptoms: first noted at 2 – 3 years of age; steady progression of weakness; limb flexion and contraction; scoliosis; dilated cardiomyopathy, conduction abnormalities, or dysrhythmias; respiratory insufficiency

  - Management: prednisone or deflazacort; monitor CO_2 levels; noninvasive ventilator support may be needed; supportive treatment of symptoms related to falls, cardiovascular disorders

- **Myasthenia gravis (MG)** is an autoimmune disorder that causes cell-mediated destruction of acetylcholine receptors, resulting in episodic muscle weakness and fatigue. **Myasthenic crisis** is an emergent condition in which MG symptoms rapidly worsen; weakening of the bulbar and respiratory muscles can cause respiratory dysfunction.
  - □ Signs and Symptoms (MG): weakened eye muscles and visual disturbances; dysphagia; fatigue; diagnosed with Tensilon (edrophonium) test
  - □ Signs and Symptoms (myasthenic crisis): dyspnea; respiratory failure; tachycardia; hypertension; no cough or gag reflex; urinary and bowel incontinence
  - □ Management: IV fluids; IV immunoglobulin; anticholinesterase (e.g., edrophonium); respiratory support

HELPFUL HINT

Patients with MG are at risk for a cholinergic crisis if they are given high doses of anticholinesterase medications.

QUICK REVIEW QUESTION

1. A patient presents to the ED with a recent diagnosis of ALS. What type of weakness would the ED nurse expect the patient to exhibit?

HEADACHES ★

Table 3.1. Diagnosis and Management of Headaches

CONDITION	TREATMENT AND MANAGEMENT
CLUSTER HEADACHES • characterized by intense unilateral pain in the periorbital or temporal area, with ipsilateral autonomic symptoms • happens at the same time each day, often waking the patient at night • episodic, lasting from 1 to 3 months, with more than 1 episode of headaches a day • can go into remission for months to years	• usually resolves within 30 minutes to 1 hour • 100% oxygen via non-rebreather • triptans (e.g., sumatriptan)
MIGRAINE • a neurovascular condition caused by neurological changes that result in vasoconstriction or vasodilation of the intracranial vessels • intense or debilitating headache (typically unilateral) lasting from 4 hours to several days • accompanied by nausea, vomiting, and sensitivity to light and sound • may be preceded by aura	• analgesics (NSAIDs) • triptans (e.g., sumatriptan) • dihydroergotamine • antiemetics • limit sensory triggers and apply ice packs to painful area

Table 3.1. Diagnosis and Management of Headaches (continued)

CONDITION	TREATMENT AND MANAGEMENT
TEMPORAL ARTERITIS • headache caused by inflamed or damaged arteries in the temporal area become inflamed or damaged • severe, throbbing headache in the temporal or forehead region, combined with scalp pain that is exacerbated with touch • muscle pain in the jaw or tongue • small period of full or partial blindness in one eye; may progress to both eyes • fever • definitive diagnostic test: biopsy of the temporal artery • rare in patients < 50 years old	• glucocorticoids (e.g., prednisone, methylprednisolone): early intervention to prevent permanent blindness • methotrexate if glucocorticoid contraindicated
TENSION HEADACHES • headaches characterized by generalized mild pain without any of the symptoms associated with migraines, such as nausea or photophobia • can be either episodic or chronic • pain is mild to moderate, often described as a vise pressing on the head • originates in the occipital or frontal area bilaterally	• NSAIDs • barbiturates or opioids (Fioricet [butalbital, acetaminophen, and caffeine] or morphine) for severe pain

DID YOU KNOW?

Post-traumatic headaches start within 7 days of a traumatic injury and typically resolve within 3 months. They may resemble migraines or tension headaches and can be treated similarly.

QUICK REVIEW QUESTION

2. A patient in the ED is diagnosed with temporal arteritis and is experiencing temporary episodes of blindness in the left eye. What intervention would the nurse anticipate?

★ INCREASED INTRACRANIAL PRESSURE

PATHOPHYSIOLOGY

INTRACRANIAL PRESSURE (ICP) is the pressure exerted on the skull and brain by the CSF in the subarachnoid space. Normal ICP values vary with age:

- Adults: 10 – 15 mm Hg
- Children: 3 – 7 mm Hg
- Term infants: 1.5 – 6 mm Hg

Increased ICP is an emergent condition that can restrict cerebral blood flow and cause permanent damage to the brain or death. Several underlying conditions can lead to increased ICP, including an increase in CSF, tumors, trauma, cerebrovascular accidents, hypertension, and infections.

DIAGNOSIS

- ICP of 20 mm Hg or higher (for adults)
- Cushing triad: bradycardia, hypertension, respiratory depression
- headache
- nausea and vomiting
- diplopia
- pupils unreactive to light
- decreased LOC
- seizures, loss of consciousness, or coma
- in patients under 12 months old: separation of bony plates or bulging fontanel

TREATMENT AND MANAGEMENT

- urgent goal is to reduce the pressure to < 20 mm Hg
- IV mannitol
- IV isotonic or hypertonic saline
- elevate head of bed to 30 degrees
- sedatives (to reduce anxiety)
- hyperventilation (PCO_2: 26 to 30 mmHg)

HELPFUL HINT

Hypotonic solutions (e.g., D5W) should not be given to patients at risk of ICP because it moves fluid from extracellular to intracellular space, increasing ICP.

QUICK REVIEW QUESTION

3. What is the normal ICP, and when is treatment for ICP usually initiated for adults?

MENINGITIS

PATHOPHYSIOLOGY

MENINGITIS is an inflammation of the meninges of the brain and spinal cord. The inflammation is caused by infections, usually viral but also bacterial, fungal, or parasitic. Acute meningitis can develop within a few days to a few weeks.

DIAGNOSIS

- stiff neck
- extremely painful to move the neck forward
- severe headache
- fever
- CSF analysis
- CBC with differential and culture to identify pathogen
- MRI or CT scan to identify inflammation in brain

TREATMENT AND MANAGEMENT

- standard and droplet isolation precautions until specific cause is determined
- IV antibiotics, antivirals, antifungal, or anti-parasitic as appropriate
- glucocorticoids
- manage ICP

QUICK REVIEW QUESTION

4. An 18-year-old college student comes into the ED complaining of a severe headache, a fever, and a stiff neck. On examination, the student is unable to turn his or her head because of stiffness and complains about extreme pain when attempting to move the head forward. What test should the nurse anticipate to prepare the patient for?

★ SEIZURE DISORDERS

PATHOPHYSIOLOGY

A SEIZURE is caused by abnormal electrical discharges in the cortical gray matter of the brain; the discharges interrupt normal brain function. TONIC-CLONIC SEIZURES start with a tonic, or contracted, state in which the patient stiffens and loses consciousness; this phase usually lasts less than 1 minute. The tonic phase is followed by the clonic phase, in which the patient's muscles rapidly contract and relax. The clonic phase can last up to several minutes.

STATUS EPILEPTICUS occurs when a seizure lasts longer than 5 minutes or when seizures occur repeatedly without a period of recovered consciousness between them.

SIGNS AND SYMPTOMS

- loss of consciousness and falling to ground
- initial contraction followed by rapid alternation between contraction and relaxation, usually lasting 1 – 2 minutes
- urinary and fecal incontinence
- status epilepticus: seizure activity lasting longer than 5 minutes or repeat seizures with no regaining of consciousness between

TREATMENT AND MANAGEMENT

- prevent injury
  - ☐ roll patient on the left side to avoid aspiration
  - ☐ loosen clothes around the neck
  - ☐ place a pillow under patient's head and remove objects near head
- manage airway

- first-line treatment: benzodiazepines (diazepam, lorazepam, or midazolam)

- second-line treatment: levetiracetam (Keppra), fosphenytoin (Cerebyx IV), valproic acid

- sedation, intubation, and mechanical ventilation when pharmacological intervention in ineffective

QUICK REVIEW QUESTION

5. A patient with a history of seizures is brought into the ED during an active tonic-clonic seizure. What medication should the nurse prepare to administer?

SHUNT DYSFUNCTIONS

PATHOPHYSIOLOGY

Hydrocephalus is treated by placing a shunt inside a brain ventricle to allow for draining of fluid from the brain into another area of the body. A shunt can malfunction when it becomes partly or fully blocked by cells, tissue, or bacterial growth. A shunt can also break down or come apart, or the valve can fail.

DIAGNOSIS

- swelling or redness along shunt tract

- headache

- vomiting

- lethargy

- irritability or confusion

- gait abnormalities or disturbances

- seizures

- urinary urgencies or incontinence

- CT scan or X-ray showing incorrect placement or blockage

TREATMENT AND MANAGEMENT

- temporary draining system is put into place until permanent shunt is reinstalled

- surgery to remove infected or malfunctioning shunt

- special pediatric considerations: abnormal head enlargement or tense, bulging fontanel

QUICK REVIEW QUESTION

6. How can the nurse assess if a pediatric patient with hydrocephalus and a shunt in place could be experiencing a shunt blockage?

SPINAL CORD INJURIES

Neurogenic Shock

PATHOPHYSIOLOGY

NEUROGENIC SHOCK is a form of shock caused by an injury or trauma to the spinal cord, typically above the level of T6. Neurogenic shock disrupts the functioning of the automatic nervous system, producing massive vasodilation.

DIAGNOSIS

- hemodynamic triad: rapid onset of hypotension, bradycardia, hypothermia
- wide pulse pressure
- skin warm, flushed, and dry
- priapism
- CT scan or MRI may show spinal cord injury

TREATMENT AND MANAGEMENT

- first-line treatment: IV fluids
- vasopressors and/or inotropes if hypotension persists
- atropine (for bradycardia)
- spine immobilization

QUICK REVIEW QUESTION

7. What characteristic of neurogenic shock is the opposite of symptoms seen in other types of shock?

Other Spinal Cord Injuries

- ANTERIOR SPINAL CORD SYNDROME occurs when the blood flow to the anterior spinal artery is disrupted, resulting in ischemia in the spinal cord; typically occurs because of hyperflexion. Signs and symptoms include complete motor loss below the lesion; loss of sensation of pain and temperature below the lesion; back or chest pain.

- BROWN-SÉQUARD SYNDROME is a spinal cord injury caused by complete cord hemitransection, typically at the cervical level. Signs and symptoms include ipsilateral motor loss below the lesion and contralateral loss of sensation of pain and temperature.

- CAUDA EQUINA SYNDROME is a spinal cord injury typically caused by compression or damage to the cauda equina (the nerve bundle that innervates the lower limbs and pelvic organs, most notably the bladder). Signs and symptoms include sensory loss in the lower extremities; bowel and bladder dysfunction; severe lower back pain; numbness in saddle area; loss of reflexes in upper extremities.

- **CENTRAL CORD SYNDROME** is caused by spinal cord compression and edema, which causes the lateral corticospinal tract white matter to deteriorate. It is the most common spinal cord injury. Signs and symptoms include greater motor function loss in the upper extremities than in the lower extremities; weakness; paresthesia in upper extremities.

- **POSTERIOR CORD SYNDROME** is a rare type of spinal cord injury caused by a lesion on the posterior spinal cord or when the spinal cord artery becomes occluded; can occur from hyperextension or a disease process. Signs and symptoms include ipsilateral loss of proprioception, vibration, fine touch, and pressure; absent deep tendon reflexes; numbness and paresthesia; paralysis.

- Management of spinal injuries: priority is ABCs; spinal immobilization; respiratory support; urinary catheter; IV fluids, vasopressors as needed for hypotension; CT scan or MRI to diagnose

- **AUTONOMIC DYSREFLEXIA** is overstimulation of the autonomic nervous system following spinal cord injuries above the T6 level. A sympathetic stimulation to the lower portion of the body leads to vasoconstriction below the area of injury, pushing blood to the upper body.
  - ☐ Signs and Symptoms: flushing and sweating above the level of injury; cold, clammy skin below the level of injury; bradycardia; sudden, severe headache; hypertension
  - ☐ Management: anti-hypertensives; treat underlying cause; have patient empty the bladder and bowel; remove tight, restrictive clothing

QUICK REVIEW QUESTION

8. A patient with a gunshot wound to the right lower back would exhibit what characteristic sign of Brown-Séquard syndrome?

STROKE ★

Hemorrhagic Stroke

PATHOPHYSIOLOGY

A **HEMORRHAGIC STROKE** occurs when a vessel ruptures in the brain or when an aneurysm bursts. The blood that accumulates in the brain leads to increased ICP and edema, which damages brain tissue and causes neurological impairment.

DIAGNOSIS

- severe, sudden headache
- sudden onset of weakness
- difficulty speaking or walking
- lethargy
- seizures

- coma
- CT scan to show location of bleed

TREATMENT AND MANAGEMENT

- manage airway
- antihypertensives
- monitor for and treat ICP
- discontinue anticoagulants and give antidotes
- possible seizure prophylaxis; benzodiazepines for seizures
- possible surgery to repair aneurysm

QUICK REVIEW QUESTION

9. What is the nursing priority for a patient admitted with a hemorrhagic stroke?

Ischemic Stroke

PATHOPHYSIOLOGY

An **ISCHEMIC STROKE** occurs when blood flow within an artery in the brain is blocked, leading to ischemia and damage to brain tissue. The lack of blood flow can be caused by a thrombosis or an embolus.

DIAGNOSIS

- facial drooping, usually on one side
- numbness, paralysis, or weakness on one side of the body
- slurred speech or inability to speak
- confusion
- vision changes
- dizziness or loss of balance control
- sudden onset of severe headache
- arm drift may be present
- CT scan without contrast to exclude hemorrhage (must be done within 25 minutes of arrival at ED)
- bedside glucose check to rule out hypoglycemia as cause of symptoms
- National Institutes of Health Stroke Scale (NIHSS) to measure patient's neurological deficits

TREATMENT AND MANAGEMENT

- tPA administered if criteria met
  - ☐ CT scan negative for hemorrhage
  - ☐ tPA should be administered within 3 – 4.5 hours of last time patient was seen normal

- tPA is contraindicated for patients with recent neurosurgery, head trauma, or stroke in previous 3 months.
- Blood pressure is strictly controlled during tPA administration; it must be kept less than 185 mm Hg systolic and less than 110 diastolic.
- monitor patient for signs of bleeding (main side effect of tPA)

HELPFUL HINT
Cardiac dysrhythmias are common post-reperfusion of occluded vessels.

- mechanical thrombectomy
- antiplatelets (aspirin) and/or anticoagulants (heparin)

QUICK REVIEW QUESTION

10. A patient presents to the ED with slurred speech and a left-sided facial droop. What is the priority for this patient?

Transient Ischemic Attack (TIA)

PATHOPHYSIOLOGY

A TRANSIENT ISCHEMIC ATTACK (TIA), a sudden, transient neurological deficit resulting from brain ischemia, does not cause permanent damage or infarction. Symptoms will vary depending on the area of the brain affected. Most TIAs last less than 5 minutes and are resolved within 1 hour. A majority are caused by emboli in the carotid or vertebral arteries.

DIAGNOSIS

- s/s of ischemic stroke, usually last less than 1 hour
- CT scan to rule out hemorrhage
- (NIHSS) to measure patient's neurological deficits

TREATMENT AND MANAGEMENT

- antiplatelets (aspirin) and/or anticoagulants (heparin)
- discharge teaching: modifying risk factors for stroke

QUICK REVIEW QUESTION

11. A patient presents to the ED with complaints of dizziness, headache, and left arm weakness. The patient says these symptoms began about 20 minutes ago and have since improved. The patient has clear speech and answers questions appropriately. What priority interventions should the nurse anticipate?

TRAUMATIC BRAIN INJURY (TBI)

- **BASILAR SKULL FRACTURE** occurs at the base of the skull in either the anterior, the middle, or the posterior fossa; the temporal bone is the most commonly affected.
  - Signs and Symptoms: Battle's sign, leakage of CSF from ears or nose, raccoon eyes, hemotympanum; impaired gag reflex; epistaxis

HELPFUL HINT
For patients with basilar skull fracture, strictly avoid placing anything in patient's nasal cavity. No nasal cannulas, nasogastric tube insertion, or nasal intubation.

□ Management: typically heal on their own without treatment; patient will be admitted for observation; monitor for and treat ICP; analgesics; surgery if CSF leakage is severe

- **BRAIN CONTUSION** is a bruise of the brain caused by closed or open head trauma. It can enlarge hours or days after the initial trauma, leading to neurological deterioration.
  - □ Signs and Symptoms: changes in LOC; memory loss; behavior changes; motor or sensory dysfunction
  - □ Management: treat hypertension and ICP; control bleeding

- **CONCUSSION** is a transient and reversible alteration in mental status following trauma to the head. Alterations can last from minutes to any time less than 6 hours.
  - □ Signs and Symptoms: temporary loss of consciousness (seconds to a few minutes); confusion or amnesia; nausea and vomiting; headache; tinnitus; visual disturbances; CT scan rarely abnormal; GCS mild (14 – 15)
  - □ Management: no treatment is usually required; analgesics; antiemetics
  - □ Discharge Teaching: rest, OTC analgesics, sleep permitted as needed

- **DIFFUSE AXONAL INJURY (DAI)** occurs when there is a widespread damage to axons in the white matter if the soft tissue of the brain rapidly accelerates or decelerates. It can also occur secondarily to an initial brain trauma because of an influx of calcium.
  - □ Signs and Symptoms: decreased or complete loss of consciousness; decorticate or decerebrate posturing; hypertension; diaphoresis; hyperthermia; amnesia; confusion; retinal hemorrhages
  - □ Management: treat hypertension and ICP; supportive treatment for symptoms

- **INTRACRANIAL HEMORRHAGE** is bleeding that occurs within the skull. They are classified as epidural, subdural, or subarachnoid depending on the location of the bleeding.
  - □ Signs and Symptoms: headache; confusion; irritability; decreased LOC; nausea and vomiting; seizures
  - □ Management: manage airway; spinal precautions; analgesics; antiemetics; treat hypertension and ICP; prepare patient for surgery

- **SECONDARY BRAIN INJURY** occurs after an initial trauma: the initial injury to the brain causes pathological changes of the endogenic neurochemical systems, resulting in secondary injury to the brain. They typically occur anywhere from 12 hours to 10 days after the injury.
  - □ Signs and Symptoms: cerebral edema, brain herniation, or cerebral ischemia; increased ICP; hypotension; hypercapnia; headache; nausea and vomiting; confusion or behavior changes
  - □ Management: treat underlying cause; respiratory support; treat hypertension and ICP; maintain normal glucose levels and body temperature

HELPFUL HINT

Headaches associated with subarachnoid hemorrhage are sudden and severe; they are often described as the worst headache of the patient's life. Patients with this type of headache should always be evaluated for intra-cranial bleeding.

DID YOU KNOW?

Any patient with a complaint of sudden, severe headache should have a subarachnoid hemorrhage ruled out as the cause.

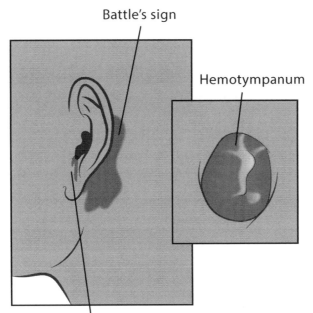

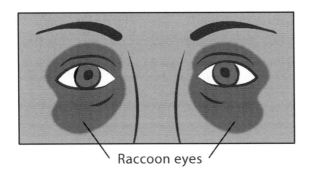

Figure 3.1. Signs of Basilar Skull Fracture

QUICK REVIEW QUESTION

12. What characteristic signs would the nurse expect to see in a patient with a basilar skull fracture?

ANSWER KEY

1. A patient with ALS presents with a progressive asymmetrical pattern of weakness that affects both upper and lower extremities.

2. The nurse should anticipate placing an IV and starting IV methylprednisolone.

3. Normal ICP is between 5 and 15 mm Hg; ICP treatment is usually initiated at 20 mm Hg or above.

4. The nurse should expect that the physician will order a lumbar puncture to collect CSF.

5. The nurse should be prepared to administer benzodiazepines, such as diazepam or lorazepam.

6. The nurse can measure the head circumference to assess if there is swelling in the cranial area.

7. A patient with neurogenic shock typically presents with warm, flushed, and dry skin as compared with other types of shock, which present with pale, cool, and clammy skin.

8. A patient with Brown-Séquard syndrome and a right-sided injury would probably experience right-sided hemiparesis and decreased pain and temperature sensation on the left side.

9. The nursing priority is to reduce blood pressure and intracranial pressure.

10. The priority intervention for a patient with a suspected ischemic stroke is to get a noncontrast CT scan of the head immediately. After the scan is completed, the ED nurse should conduct a bedside glucose check, place an IV, and draw labs.

11. The nurse should suspect that the patient has had a TIA, in light of symptom presentation. The nurse would anticipate a complete stroke workup, including CT scan of the head, NIHSS, IV placement, lab draw, and admission.

12. The nurse would expect to see raccoon eyes, Battle's sign, hemotympanum, otorrhea, and rhinorrhea in a patient with a basilar skull fracture.

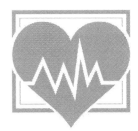

4

GASTROINTESTINAL EMERGENCIES

BCEN CONTENT OUTLINE

* **A. ACUTE ABDOMEN** (e.g., peritonitis, appendicitis)
* **B. BLEEDING**
* **C. CHOLECYSTITIS**
  D. Cirrhosis
* **E. DIVERTICULITIS**
  F. Esophageal varices
  G. Esophagitis
  H. Foreign bodies
  I. Gastritis
* **J. GASTROENTERITIS**
  K. Hepatitis
  L. Hernia
  M. Inflammatory bowel disease
  N. Intussusception
  O. Obstructions
* **P. PANCREATITIS**
  Q. Trauma
  R. Ulcers

ACUTE ABDOMEN ✶

ACUTE ABDOMEN is sudden, severe abdominal pain. The physical examination of patients with acute abdomen should focus on pain location, history of GI symptoms, and palpitation to assess for rigidity or guarding. Cardiovascular, genitourinary, and obstetrical conditions should also be considered when assessing acute abdomen.

Table 4.1. Causes of Acute Abdomen

CONDITION	PATHOPHYSIOLOGY	SYMPTOMS
Abdominal aortic aneurysm (AAA)	widening of the aorta in the abdomen	sharp, severe pain in the chest, back, abdomen, or flank; rapid, weak, or absent pulse; hypotension
Appendicitis	inflammation of the appendix	RLQ pain; rebound tenderness; positive psoas sign; fever
Cholecystitis	inflammation of the gallbladder	colicky RUQ pain, which can radiate to back or right shoulder; positive Murphy's sign
Kidney stones	blockage in the urethra leading to inflammation of the kidney	unilateral flank pain (can be severe); hematuria
Pancreatitis	inflammation of the pancreas	upper abdominal and back pain; distension of abdomen
Peptic ulcer	erosion of the stomach by stomach acid	upper abdomen and back pain; heartburn
Ruptured ectopic pregnancy	rupture of the fallopian tube due to ectopic pregnancy	vaginal bleeding, abdominal pain, cessation of pregnancy s/s
Ruptured ovarian cyst	rupture of cyst in the ovary	sudden, severe, unilateral pelvic pain

QUICK REVIEW QUESTION

1. During assessment of a patient with acute abdomen, the nurse notes right lower quadrant pain, rebound tenderness, and positive psoas sign. What condition should the nurse suspect?

BLEEDING

Upper GI Bleeding

PATHOPHYSIOLOGY

An UPPER GI BLEED is bleeding that occurs between the esophagus and duodenum. Bleeding may be severe and require immediate hemodynamic management. Etiology of the bleeding varies:

- PEPTIC ULCERS and ESOPHAGITIS (secondary to GERD) are the most common causes of upper GI bleeding.

- ESOPHAGEAL VARICES occur when veins in the esophagus rupture because of portal hypertension (usually caused by hepatic cirrhosis). Bleeding may be severe and is likely to recur.

- ESOPHAGEAL PERFORATION or RUPTURE may be iatrogenic, secondary to trauma, or caused by the severe effort of vomiting (BOERHAAVE SYNDROME).

- **MALLORY-WEISS TEARS** occur at the gastroesophageal junction and result from forceful vomiting.
- NSAIDs and chronic gastritis can cause or worsen upper GI bleeding.

DIAGNOSIS

- upper abdominal pain
- hematemesis (may be in nasogastric aspirate)
- melena
- coffee-ground emesis
- hematochezia (if hemorrhaging)
- signs and symptoms of hypovolemia (after significant blood loss)
- decreased HgB, Hct, and platelets
- longer PT and aPTT
- elevated BUN and BUN:creatinine ratio
- positive hemoccult
- diagnosed via appropriate endoscopy or angiogram (EGD to locate source of bleeding)

HELPFUL HINT
Elevated BUN:creatinine ratio is associated with decreased kidney function and increased breakdown of protein. It is often seen with upper GI bleeds (due to digestion of blood) but not with lower GI bleeds.

TREATMENT AND MANAGEMENT

- oxygen as needed
- manage hemodynamic status: IV fluids, blood products, and management of coagulopathies
- medications to constrict vasculature: vasopressin, octreotides (e.g., Sandostatin), and beta blockers
- endoscopic or surgical repair if bleeding persists

QUICK REVIEW QUESTION

2. The physician has ordered an octreotide drip for a patient diagnosed with esophageal varices. The nurse knows that this medication is appropriate for this diagnosis because it has what type of action?

Lower GI Bleeding

PATHOPHYSIOLOGY

A **LOWER GI BLEED** is any bleeding that occurs below the duodenum. Lower GI bleeds occur less frequently than do upper GI bleeds, are typically less emergent, and may stop on their own. They are usually caused by disease or tumors in the colon.

DIAGNOSIS

- abdominal or chest pain
- hematochezia

- melena

- bleeding from rectum

- signs and symptoms of hypovolemia (after significant blood loss)

- positive hemoccult

- decreased HgB and Hct

- PT and aPTT may be longer

- diagnosed via appropriate endoscopy, CT scan, or angiogram

TREATMENT AND MANAGEMENT

- manage hemodynamic status: IV fluids, blood products, and management of coagulopathies

- endoscopic or surgical repair if bleeding persists

QUICK REVIEW QUESTION

3. What signs and symptoms would the critical care nurse expect to see in a patient with a lower GI bleed?

CIRRHOSIS

LIVER FAILURE can be acute (onset < 26 weeks) or chronic. Common causes of acute liver failure (also called FULMINATE HEPATITIS) include acetaminophen overdose and viral hepatitis; the most common cause of chronic liver failure is alcohol abuse.

Liver failure leads to dysfunction in multiple organ systems.

- **HEPATIC ENCEPHALOPATHY** is impaired cognitive function caused by increased serum ammonia (NH_3) levels. NH_3 is produced by bacteria in the bowels and is normally broken down by healthy liver tissue before it enters circulation.

- Increased NH_3 levels may also cause neuromuscular symptoms, including asterixis and bradykinesia.

- Coagulopathies are caused by impaired synthesis of clotting factors in liver tissue.

- **JAUNDICE** is caused by hyperbilirubinemia.

- Acute kidney injury occurs in approximately 50% of patients with liver failure (the mechanism is unknown).

- Infections and sepsis develop secondary to decreased and defective WBCs.

- Metabolic imbalances may include hypokalemia, hyponatremia, and hypoglycemia.

- Lowered peripheral vascular resistance decreases BP and increases HR.

Chronic liver failure leads to CIRRHOSIS—the development of fibrotic tissue in the liver. Cirrhosis in the liver increases resistance in the portal vein, causing

PORTAL HYPERTENSION. Common conditions that occur secondary to portal hypertension include esophageal varices, ASCITES, and SPLENOMEGALY.

DIAGNOSIS

- cognitive changes or motor dysfunction
- jaundice
- petechiae or purpura
- spider angiomas
- ascites
- RUQ pain
- palmar erythema
- nausea and vomiting
- elevated AST, ALT, and/or bilirubin
- elevated NH_3 levels
- decreased protein, albumin, and fibrinogen
- decreased WBCs, HgB, Hct, and platelets
- longer PT and PTT, and increased INR
- CT scan or MRI may show fibrosis of liver

HELPFUL HINT
Sedatives should be used cautiously in patients with liver failure because of the liver's inability to clear them. Low doses of short-acting benzodiazepines should be used when sedation is necessary.

TREATMENT AND MANAGEMENT

- fluid resuscitation
- lactulose and neomycin to reduce ammonia levels
- diuretics (e.g., spironolactone) for ascites
- prophylactic treatment for stress ulcers
- corticosteroids and antiviral medications for viral infections
- monitor ICP
- alcohol withdrawal protocols if indicated (See Ch. 15, "Toxicology Emergencies" for more information on alcohol withdrawal.)
- tight glucose control for nonalcoholic fatty liver disease

QUICK REVIEW QUESTION

4. A nurse is providing care to a patient with acute liver failure. What should the nurse expect to see in the patient's CBC and coagulation tests?

GI INFLAMMATION ★

- **APPENDICITIS** is inflammation of the appendix; obstruction of the appendiceal lumen results in a decrease in blood supply which can lead to necrosis and perforation.

- Diagnosis: dull, steady periumbilical pain; RLQ pain that worsens with movement; pain in RLQ at McBurney's point; positive Rovsing's sign; positive psoas sign; fever; nausea and vomiting; abdominal rigidity and rebound tenderness; CT scan to diagnose
- Management: antiemetics; analgesics; keep patient NPO and prep for surgery

- **CHOLECYSTITIS** is acute or chronic inflammation of the gallbladder, usually resulting from an impacted stone in the neck of the gallbladder or in the cystic duct.
  - Diagnosis: colicky RUQ pain, which can radiate to back or right shoulder; positive Murphy's sign; nausea, vomiting, or flatulence; jaundice if obstruction is significant; CT or ultrasound to diagnose
  - Management: analgesics; antiemetics; ERCP to remove stones in bile duct; laparoscopic removal of gallbladder for rupture or liver/pancreas damage

- **DIVERTICULITIS** is inflammation of the diverticula (small outpouchings in the GI tract, usually in the sigmoid colon); the inflammation can cause necrosis and perforation.

  - Diagnosis: LLQ abdominal pain; abdominal distention and rebound tenderness; nausea and vomiting; fever; diarrhea or constipation; hematochezia
  - Management: antibiotics; electrolytes as needed; liquid diet
  - Discharge teaching: stool softeners; liquid diet followed by a low-fiber diet until the inflammation is reduced, then a high-fiber diet

- **ESOPHAGITIS** is an inflammation of the esophagus, usually secondary to GERD.
  - Diagnosis: burning pain within an hour of eating; sore throat; pain worsens with increased intra-abdominal pressure (bending, sneezing, lying flat)
  - Management: antacid, lidocaine, and anticholinergic (GI "cocktail"); proton pump inhibitors or H2 blockers
  - Discharge teaching: lifestyle changes to reduce reflux

- **GASTRITIS** is the inflammation or irritation of the stomach lining.
  - Diagnosis: epigastric pain; nausea and vomiting; diarrhea; poor appetite; positive H. pylori infection
  - Management: antiemetics; H2 blocker or PPI; antacid; electrolyte and fluid replacement
  - Discharge teaching: lifestyle changes to reduce reflux

- **GASTROENTERITIS** is inflammation of the stomach and intestines due to bacterial, viral, or parasitic infection. Onset of symptoms is rapid.
  - Diagnosis: nausea, vomiting, or diarrhea; diffuse and cramping abdominal pain; fever; dehydration; hyperactive bowel sounds; labs consistent with dehydration
  - Management: electrolyte and fluid replacement; antiemetics; anticholinergics

- Discharge teaching: BRAT diet
- **HEPATITIS** is inflammation of the liver. It can be caused by a systemic viral infection, autoimmune conditions, or by certain medications, including acetaminophen, niacin, IV amiodarone, IV methotrexate, and chemotherapy drugs.
  - Diagnosis: clay-colored stools; dark urine (foamy); jaundice; steatorrhea; flulike symptoms; abdominal pain; elevated liver enzymes (AST and ALT), alkaline phosphatase, and ammonia; low albumin
  - Management: lactulose for elevated ammonia levels; treatment for underlying condition (e.g., antivirals, antidotes)
- **PERITONITIS** is inflammation of the peritoneum (the lining of the abdominal cavity) caused by a blood-borne organism or from the perforation of an organ.
  - Diagnosis: rigid abdomen; fever; diffuse pain that worsens with movement and is relieved by flexing the knees or bending right hip; guarding of abdomen; rebound tenderness; positive Markle test; labs show infection
  - Management: broad-spectrum antibiotics; antiemetics; analgesics; keep patient NPO and prep for surgery

QUICK REVIEW QUESTION

5. A patient presents to the ED with RLQ pain, nausea, and vomiting. The patient is diagnosed with appendicitis. What priority interventions should the nurse prepare for?

FOREIGN BODIES IN THE GI SYSTEM

PATHOPHYSIOLOGY

A **FOREIGN BODY** is any object that enters the GI system either intentionally or accidently. Foreign bodies within the GI system typically present as partial or full obstructions of the esophagus, although objects may also pass to other GI organs. These objects can cause damage, including tears, infection, and obstruction, to the GI system.

DIAGNOSIS

- drooling or difficulty swallowing
- feeling of something "stuck" in throat
- subcutaneous emphysema present if esophageal perforation
- chest or neck X-rays to diagnose

TREATMENT AND MANAGEMENT

- maintain airway
- glucagon to promote smooth muscle relaxation
- endoscopy or surgery to remove objects that don't pass on their own

6. A patient presents to triage with complaints of feeling as if something is lodged in her throat after eating dinner. What is the priority intervention for a patient?

HERNIA

PATHOPHYSIOLOGY

A **HERNIA** occurs when a portion of the abdominal contents protrudes through the abdominal wall. Common areas for hernias are epigastric, umbilical, inguinal, and femoral. To determine treatment, medical personnel must determine whether the hernia has a good blood supply or is **INCARCERATED** (trapped).

Incarcerated inguinal hernias may become strangulated (cut off from blood supply), resulting in ischemia in the trapped tissue. An **INCARCERATED INGUINAL HERNIA** with ischemia is an emergent condition that can lead to bowel necrosis, sepsis, and neurogenic shock.

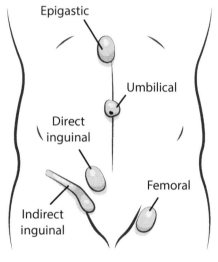

Figure 4.1. Common Hernia Locations

DIAGNOSIS

- pain at hernia site
- swelling at hernia site, usually a firm, tender mass
- nausea and vomiting
- strangulation hernia
  - □ tachycardia
  - □ abdominal distention
  - □ fever
- CT scan to diagnose incarceration

TREATMENT AND MANAGEMENT

- no incarceration: hernia is manually reduced
- incarcerated or cannot be reduced: prep patient for surgery

QUICK REVIEW QUESTION

7. A patient arrives at the ED and says he believes he has a hernia. What assessments can the ED nurse perform to confirm?

INFLAMMATORY BOWEL DISEASE

- **CROHN'S DISEASE** is a chronic inflammatory bowel disease. It can involve any part of the GI tract, but most commonly occurs in the small or large intestine.
    - ☐ Diagnosis: loose stools (5 – 6 episodes per day); abdominal pain, typically described as cramping and continuous; steatorrhea; fever; weight loss; associated anal fissures or abscesses; endoscopy for diagnosis
    - ☐ Management: keep patient NPO; immunosuppressants (e.g., infliximab [Remicade]); corticosteroids

- **ULCERATIVE COLITIS** is a type of inflammatory bowel disease that involves the large colon. The intestines become inflamed, and patients typically have exacerbations and remissions.
    - ☐ Diagnosis: hematochezia (10 – 20 episodes per day); weight loss; fever; cramping, abdominal pain, typically in the LLQ; dehydration
    - ☐ Management: fluids; anti-inflammatories; corticosteroids

QUICK REVIEW QUESTION

8. A patient arrives at the ED with complaints of frequent bloody stools. What further assessment findings would the ED nurse expect to find in a patient diagnosed with ulcerative colitis?

INTUSSUSCEPTION

PATHOPHYSIOLOGY

INTUSSUSCEPTION is a mechanical bowel obstruction caused when a loop of the large intestine *telescopes* within itself. This condition can cut off the blood supply, causing perforation, infection, and bowel ischemia. It usually occurs within the first 3 years of life and is more prevalent in males.

DIAGNOSIS

- red currant-jelly–like stool
- sausage-shaped abdominal mass
- colicky pain
- inconsolable crying
- absence of stools
- abdominal X-rays to confirm diagnosis

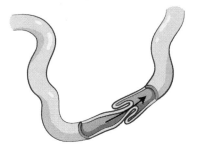

Figure 4.2. Intussusception

TREATMENT AND MANAGEMENT

- keep patient NPO
- barium enema: the weight of the barium helps push the telescoped bowel out

9. A 10-month-old infant patient presents to the ED with persistent crying and red stool with a gelatinous consistency. What condition and treatment does the ED nurse suspect?

BOWEL OBSTRUCTION

PATHOPHYSIOLOGY

A **BOWEL OBSTRUCTION** occurs when normal flow through the bowel is disrupted. **MECHANICAL OBSTRUCTIONS** are physical barriers in the bowel. The most common mechanical obstructions in the small bowel are **ADHESIONS**, **HERNIAS**, and **VOLVULUS** (twisting of the bowels). The most common obstruction in the large bowel are tumors.

PARALYTIC ILEUS is the impairment of peristalsis in the absence of mechanical obstruction. It is most common in postoperative patients and can also be caused by endocrine disorders or medications (e.g., opioids).

Increased pressure proximal to the obstruction can lead to **PERFORATION** of the bowel wall. Other common causes of bowel perforation include surgery, abdominal trauma, and neoplasm (in large bowel).

DIAGNOSIS

- nausea and vomiting
- diarrhea
- distended and firm abdomen
- abdominal pain (cramping and colicky)
- unable to pass flatus
- high-pitched bowel sounds (early); absent bowel sounds (late)
- tympanic percussion
- pain, often sudden onset (perforation)
- abdominal X-ray may show dilated bowel loops
- CT scan to diagnose

TREATMENT AND MANAGEMENT

- keep patient NPO
- fluid resuscitation
- antibiotics as needed
- medications for GI s/s: antiemetics, simethicone, and/or magnesium hydroxide
- surgical intervention for obstructions that do not resolve within 48 hours
- surgical closure of perforation

HELPFUL HINT

Bowel infarction (necrosis of the intestinal wall) occurs when decreased blood flow causes ischemia in the bowels. It is most commonly caused by a thromboembolism in the intestinal arteries but can occur secondary to mechanical bowel obstructions.

HELPFUL HINT

Bariatric surgeries are performed to resect, bypass, or band the stomach to promote weight loss. Common complications of bariatric bypass surgery include malabsorption, bowel obstruction, anastomotic leaks, and GI bleeding.

10. A patient presents with abdominal pain, nausea, and vomiting. A bowel obstruction is suspected and then confirmed by CT scan. What priority interventions should the nurse anticipate for this patient?

PANCREATITIS ★

PATHOPHYSIOLOGY

PANCREATITIS is caused by the release of digestive enzymes into the tissues of the pancreas. The condition causes autodigestion, inflammation, tissue destruction, and injury to adjacent structures and organs. Pancreatitis can be acute or chronic, but its onset is usually sudden. The most common causes of pancreatitis are gallstones and alcohol abuse.

The tissue damage caused by pancreatitis results in fluid shifts into interstitial spaces, leading to edema and systemic inflammatory responses (e.g., ARDS). Inflammation may also limit diaphragm movement and cause atelectasis. Severe damage to the pancreas may cause retroperitoneal bleeding.

HELPFUL HINT

Signs and symptoms of retroperitoneal bleeding (or hematoma) include hypotension; bradycardia; Grey Turner's sign; and abdominal, back, or flank pain.

DIAGNOSIS

- steady, severe pain abdominal pain; usually in the LUQ and may radiate to the back or shoulder
- guarding
- nausea and vomiting
- decreased bowel sounds
- steatorrhea
- fever
- tachycardia and hypotension
- dyspnea
- Cullen's sign
- Grey Turner's sign
- elevated amylase and lipase
- hypoglycemia
- elevated Hct, BUN, and CRP
- increased WBCs
- imaging (MRI or CT scan with contrast) to diagnose

TREATMENT AND MANAGEMENT

- fluid resuscitation, including electrolyte replacement
- pain management (usually opioids)
- keep patient NPO

- endoscopic retrograde cholangiopancreatography (ERCP) for gallstones and bile duct inflammation
- monitor for respiratory complications, including ARDS and atelectasis

QUICK REVIEW QUESTION

11. The nurse is caring for a patient who is complaining of sudden, severe abdominal pain in the mid-epigastric area that spreads to the left shoulder. What complications should the nurse assess for?

GASTROINTESTINAL TRAUMA

PATHOPHYSIOLOGY

GI TRAUMA can be caused by a penetrating injury such as a gunshot or knife wound or can be caused by blunt trauma from a motor vehicle injury or a fall.

DIAGNOSIS

Table 4.2. Diagnosis of GI Trauma

ORGAN	SIGNS AND SYMPTOMS	DIAGNOSTIC TESTS AND FINDINGS
Spleen Most frequently injured abdominal organ	• LUQ pain (referred to left shoulder) • LUQ bruising • Distended abdomen	CT scan or FAST exam may show splenic rupture
Liver Largest abdominal organ; injury most frequently caused by blunt trauma	• RUQ pain (referred to right shoulder) • RUQ bruising • Rigid abdomen • Labs consistent with liver damage	CT scan may show laceration or hemorrhage
Pancreas Most frequently missed abdominal injury with a high mortality rate	• Epigastric pain • Rebound tenderness • Elevated pancreatic enzymes	• CT for diagnosis • Testing for elevated pancreatic enzymes can be delayed in bloodwork up to 6 hours
Stomach Most commonly caused by a penetrating injury	• Hematemesis • Rigid abdomen • Rebound tenderness	Free air on chest X-ray

TREATMENT AND MANAGEMENT

- fluids/blood products for hypovolemia
- surgery required for penetration injuries and unstable patients

12. A patient is brought to the ED following a car accident. She reports acute pain in her right upper quadrant and right shoulder, and the nurse notes a rigid abdomen during the physical examination. The patient's HR is 105, and her BP is 85/60. What intervention should the nurse anticipate?

ULCERS

PATHOPHYSIOLOGY

An ULCER is a sore or opening that occurs within the stomach lining (gastric ulcer), duodenum (duodenal ulcer), esophagus, or small intestine. PEPTIC ULCERS include both gastric and duodenal ulcers. Duodenal ulcers, which cause the stomach to empty rapidly, are the most common type of ulcer. Risk factors for ulcers include frequent use of NSAIDs, or a history of NSAID use, stress, and H. pylori infection.

DIAGNOSIS

- pain described as squeezing or tightness, and may radiate to back
- burning abdominal and/or throat pain
- pain may be accompanied by bloating and a feeling of fullness
- pain either relieved or worsened by food
- duodenal ulcer: pain starts before meals; typically relieved by food
- gastric ulcer: pain chronic; occurs while eating
- endoscopy (esophagogastroduodenoscopy, or EGD) to diagnose

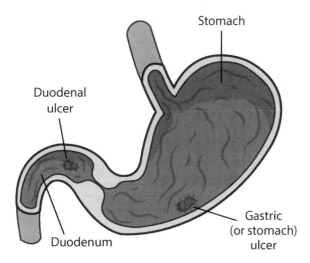

Figure 4.3. Peptic Ulcers

TREATMENT AND MANAGEMENT

- H$_2$ blockers or proton-pump inhibitors
- discharge teaching: lifestyle changes to reduce reflux

13. A patient presents to the ED with squeezing and burning abdominal and throat pain. The patient is diagnosed with an ulcer. What information should the ED nurse implement within the discharge teaching for this patient?

ANSWER KEY

1. The patient has s/s of appendicitis.

2. Because octreotide is a vasoconstrictor, it constricts the dilated vessels present in esophageal varices and reduces bleeding.

3. Early signs of a lower GI bleed include hematochezia, abdominal pain, and fatigue. Decreased HgB, decreased Hct, tachycardia, and hypotension may occur after a significant amount of blood loss and would be seen as late signs of a lower GI bleed.

4. Patients with liver failure will be pancytopenic with low levels of RBCs, platelets, and WBCs. They will also have prolonged PT and PTT, an increased INR, and low fibrinogen.

5. Priority interventions for a patient with appendicitis should be keeping the patient NPO and prepping them for surgery. The patient may be administered antiemetics, analgesics, and antibiotics before surgery.

6. The patient's airway should always be assessed first. It should be assessed for patency, and the nurse should look for signs of airway obstruction, including drooling, the inability to handle secretions, an ineffective cough, and/or stridor.

7. A full abdominal assessment should be performed to look for a bulge, mass, and/or swelling. The nurse should also gather information about the patient's activities that would cause straining, such as weightlifting. Additionally, a CT scan is necessary to rule out an incarcerated hernia.

8. In addition to hematochezia (up to 20 episodes per day), patients with ulcerative colitis may also have symptoms such as weight loss, fever, tachycardia, and cramping LLQ abdominal pain. Additionally, signs of dehydration may be present because of fluid loss from diarrhea.

9. Red jelly-like stools, along with a sausage-shaped abdominal mass, are hallmarks of intussusception. Intussusception causes the bowel to telescope into itself. A barium enema will help to push the bowel out.

10. Patients with bowel obstructions need IV fluids. During a bowel obstruction, severe vomiting and fluid sequestration in the bowel lumen lead to hypovolemia and electrolyte imbalances.

11. The patient has symptoms of acute pancreatitis. Atelectasis and other respiratory problems are common in patients with acute pancreatitis. The nurse should thoroughly assess lung sounds and note any adventitious or diminished breath sounds, look for signs of orthopnea or other dyspnea, and monitor oxygen saturation levels.

12. The patient has s/s of liver damage and is hemodynamically unstable. The nurse should anticipate the patient will require immediate surgery.

13. A patient with an ulcer should be taught to make lifestyle changes to reduce reflux. These changes may include avoid NSAIDs, smoking, alcohol, and spicy foods.

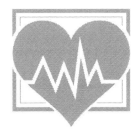

5

GENITOURINARY EMERGENCIES

BCEN CONTENT OUTLINE

    A. Foreign bodies

✯ **B. INFECTION** (e.g., urinary tract infection, pyelonephritis, epididymitis, orchitis, STDs)

    C. Priapism

✯ **D. RENAL CALCULI**

    E. Testicular torsion

    F. Trauma

    G. Urinary retention

FOREIGN BODIES IN THE GENITOURINARY SYSTEM

PATHOPHYSIOLOGY

The most common sources of foreign bodies in the genitourinary system are sexual activity, trauma, or medical intervention. The method used for removal will be based on the patient's age and the object's motility and size.

DIAGNOSIS

- urinary symptoms (e.g., hematuria, dysuria)
- lower abdominal or genital pain
- dyspareunia
- acute cystitis
- urethral discharge
- s/s of infection

DID YOU KNOW?

In female patients, larger objects may cause injury to the bladder.

- visualization of foreign body during exam
- X-ray or ultrasound showing presence of foreign body

TREATMENT AND MANAGEMENT

- analgesics as needed
- first line: remove foreign object endoscopically
- surgery if object cannot be removed endoscopically
- psychiatric consult if warranted

QUICK REVIEW QUESTION

1. A female patient presents to the ED with complaints of acute urinary retention. She reports that her partner was using a pencil to stimulate her the night before while they were both highly intoxicated. A bedside ultrasound reveals that part of the pencil is lodged in her urethra and has entered the bladder. What intervention should the nurse prepare for?

★ INFECTION

- **EPIDIDYMITIS** is inflammation of the epididymis. It is usually the result of a bacterial infection secondary to a UTI or sexually transmitted disease.
  - □ Diagnosis: gradual onset pain posterior to testes; s/s lower UTI; positive Prehn's sign; swelling and tenderness in testis; ultrasound showing enlarged epididymis; labs show infection
  - □ Management: antibiotics; pain management (analgesics, ice packs, scrotal support or elevation); epididymectomy for severe infection
- **ORCHITIS** is inflammation of the testes usually caused by a bacterial or viral infection. It can occur secondary to epididymitis (epididymo-orchitis).

DID YOU KNOW?

Mumps is the most common cause of viral orchitis.

  - □ Diagnosis: unilateral, sudden onset of pain in testis; swelling and tenderness in testis; when associated with mumps, will appear 4 – 7 days after s/s of infection; ultrasound showing increased blood flow to the affected testis
  - □ Management: antibiotics; anti-inflammatories; pain management (analgesics, ice packs, scrotal support or elevation)
- **PROSTATITIS** is inflammation of the prostate, usually caused by bacterial infection (*E. coli*). Asymptomatic cases are often discovered during unrelated assessments and are not usually treated.
  - □ Diagnosis: urinary symptoms (e.g., frequent, urgent urination; dysuria); suprapubic, perineal, or low back pain; s/s of infection; labs show infection
  - □ Management: antibiotics; analgesics
- **PYELONEPHRITIS** is infection of the kidneys. Symptoms can develop over hours or days, with some patients waiting weeks before seeking care.

- □ Diagnosis: clinical triad (fever, nausea and vomiting, costovertebral pain); cloudy, dark, foul-smelling urine; hematuria; dysuria; suprapubic, cervical, or uterine tenderness; urinalysis shows infection
- □ Management: IV fluids (D5W); antibiotics; analgesics; antipyretics; antiemetics
- A URINARY TRACT INFECTION (**UTI**) is infection in the lower urinary tract (bladder and urethra) or in the upper urinary tract (kidneys and ureters).
  - □ Diagnosis: frequent small amounts of urine; cloudy, dark, foul-smelling urine; hematuria; dysuria; pelvic, suprapubic, abdominal, or lower back pain or pressure; s/s of infection; altered mental status in patients > 65 years old; urinalysis shows infection
  - □ Management: antibiotics; supportive treatment for symptoms

QUICK REVIEW QUESTION

2. What is the clinical triad associated with pyelonephritis?

PRIAPISM

PRIAPISM is an unintentional, prolonged erection that is unrelated to sexual stimulation and is unrelieved by ejaculation. ISCHEMIC (LOW-FLOW) PRIAPISM occurs when blood becomes trapped in the erect penis. NONISCHEMIC (HIGH-FLOW) PRIAPISM is the unregulated circulation of blood through the penis resulting from a ruptured artery in the penis or perineum. Ischemic priapism is considered a medical emergency requiring immediate intervention to preserve function of the penis.

DIAGNOSIS

- ischemic priapism: rigid, painful erection unrelated to sexual activity lasting > 4 hours
- nonischemic priapism:
  - □ recurrent episodes of persistent erections (may be partial)
  - □ difficulty maintaining full erection
  - □ no pain
  - □ trauma (usually straddle injury)
  - □ delay between injury and priapism
- ultrasound showing obstructed or decreased blood flow
- venous blood gas dark or black

TREATMENT AND MANAGEMENT

- ischemic priapism: blood should be drained from the penis within 4 – 6 hours to prevent permanent damage.
  - □ first-line treatment: aspiration with intracavernosal phenylephrine injection

- □ second-line treatment: a shunt (T-shunt, Al-Ghorab's shunt, or Ebbehoj's shunt)
- □ penile prostheses for priapism lasting > 36 hours
- ◼ nonischemic priapism: the condition will often spontaneously resolve
  - □ monitor
  - □ first-line treatment, if needed: elective arterial embolization

QUICK REVIEW QUESTION

3. A 22-year-old patient in the ED is diagnosed with nonischemic priapism resulting from a straddle injury and is currently under observation. The patient is becoming increasingly anxious and tells the nurse he wants to be treated so he won't lose function in his penis. How should the nurse explain to the patient why he is not receiving medical intervention?

RENAL CALCULI

PATHOPHYSIOLOGY

RENAL CALCULI (kidney stones) are hardened mineral deposits (most often calcareous) that form in the kidneys. Renal calculi are usually asymptomatic but will cause debilitating pain and urinary symptoms once they pass into the urinary tract, where they are referred to as urinary calculi.

DIAGNOSIS

- ◼ severe, sharp, intermittent flank pain
- ◼ urinary symptoms (e.g., dysuria, hematuria)
- ◼ s/s of infection
- ◼ CT scan to diagnose calculi

TREATMENT AND MANAGEMENT

- ◼ small stones (< 5 mm) with minimal symptoms
  - □ will pass spontaneously
  - □ analgesics
  - □ alpha blockers (can help the stone pass)
  - □ encourage fluids
- ◼ large stones (> 5 mm) with symptoms: surgical intervention

QUICK REVIEW QUESTION

4. A patient presents to the ED with complaints of bloody urine and severe side and back pain. What imaging study should the nurse anticipate will be ordered?

HELPFUL HINT

Medications that may cause renal calculi include topiramate (Topamax), ciprofloxacin, sulfa antibiotics, diuretics, and decongestants.

TESTICULAR TORSION

PATHOPHYSIOLOGY

TESTICULAR TORSION occurs when the spermatic cord, which supplies blood to the testicles, becomes twisted, leading to an ischemic testicle. The condition is considered a medical emergency that requires immediate treatment to preserve the function of the testicle. Most testicular torsion cases are caused by BELL-CLAPPER DEFORMITY, in which the testicle is not correctly attached to the tunica vaginalis.

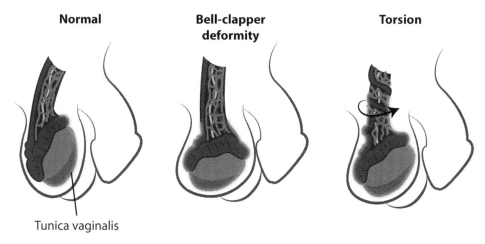

Figure 5.1. Testicular Torsion

DIAGNOSIS

- sudden, severe unilateral scrotal pain
- high-riding testicle
- absent cremasteric reflex
- signs of inflammation in scrotal skin
- ultrasound showing reduced or absent blood flow to affected testicle

TREATMENT AND MANAGEMENT

- analgesics
- prep for immediate exploratory surgery

QUICK REVIEW QUESTION

5. What is the primary risk factor for testicular torsion?

GENITOURINARY TRAUMA

PATHOPHYSIOLOGY

GENITOURINARY (GU) TRAUMA can cause injury to the kidneys, bladder, urethra, or external genitalia. GU trauma symptoms can be nonspecific and can be masked by or related to other injuries. Trauma may occur from blunt or penetrating injury.

- Renal: The majority of renal trauma occurs from blunt trauma such as direct impact into the seatbelt or steering wheel in frontal MVCs or from body panel intrusion in side-impact crashes.

- Bladder: The majority of bladder trauma occurs from blunt trauma, usually occurring with a pelvic fracture. Bladder rupture can result from lap belt restraint.

- Urethral: Urethral injuries are more common in males and may result from trauma and pelvic fracture or from iatrogenic injuries resulting from catheterization.

- External genitalia: These injuries are more common in males due to anatomical presentation and greater participation in physical sports, acts of violence, and war. Up to two-thirds of all genitourinary traumas involve the external genitalia. Injuries to the penis and scrotum may occur from use of penile rings or other sexual pleasure devices, mutilation, or straddle injuries.

DID YOU KNOW?
Penile fractures occur when there is a rupture of tissue within the penis, usually as a result of abrupt bending of the erect penis. Patient presents with penile deformity and will require surgery.

DIAGNOSIS

- pain (suprapubic, abdominal, groin/genital, or flank)
- urinary symptoms (e.g., dysuria, hematuria)
- bleeding at meatus
- ecchymosis and edema
- distended bladder or abdominal distention
- visible wound, penetration injury, or embedded object
- urinalysis, CT scan, ultrasound to diagnose injury

TREATMENT AND MANAGEMENT

- oxygen and IV fluids as needed
- analgesics
- blunt injuries: supportive care with bed rest and observation
- penetrating injuries: surgical intervention

QUICK REVIEW QUESTION

6. A 16-year-old patient presents to the ED with complaints of nausea and genital pain after sustaining a straddle injury on a skateboard. What further signs and symptoms should the nurse assess to diagnose genitourinary trauma?

URINARY RETENTION

PATHOPHYSIOLOGY

URINARY RETENTION is the inability to void the bladder. The condition can be acute or chronic and is most often caused by either an obstruction (e.g., prostatic hyperplasia, organ prolapse) or an infection (e.g., prostatitis, vulvovaginitis). Acute urinary retention is a medical emergency that can result in bladder injuries, kidney infections, and sepsis if left untreated.

DIAGNOSIS

- inability to urinate
- urinary frequency or urgency
- pelvic pressure or pain
- renal/bladder ultrasound or CT scan to identify cause of retention

TREATMENT AND MANAGEMENT

- priority intervention: immediate voiding of bladder via catheter
- treatment for underlying cause of retention after bladder is voided

QUICK REVIEW QUESTION

7. A patient in the ED states that he has not voided for 16 hours, and a bladder scan shows 600 ml of urine in the bladder. What is the nurse's priority?

ANSWER KEY

1. The nurse should prepare the patient for endoscopic removal of the object.

2. The clinical triad consists of fever, nausea and/or vomiting, and costovertebral pain.

3. The nurse should explain that during episodes of nonischemic priapism, blood continues to move through the penis and the chance of permanent damage is very low. The nurse should further explain that this type of priapism usually resolves on its own but that treatment options are available if it does not.

4. The patient has symptoms of urinary calculi. A CT scan is the preferred imaging study to visualize the location, size, and composition of the calculi.

5. Bell-clapper deformity, a genetic condition in which the testicles are not attached to the scrotum, is found in 90 percent of testicular torsion cases.

6. Common symptoms of straddle injuries, in addition to nausea and genital pain, include suprapubic or abdominal pain and dysuria.

7. The nurse should assist the patient with voiding by placing a straight catheter or a Foley catheter.

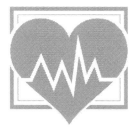

6

GYNECOLOGICAL EMERGENCIES

BCEN CONTENT OUTLINE

- ★ **A. Bleeding/dysfunction** (vaginal)
- B. Foreign bodies
- C. Hemorrhage
- ★ **D. Infection** (e.g., discharge, pelvic inflammatory disease, STDs)
- E. Ovarian cyst
- F. Sexual assault/battery
- G. Trauma

BLEEDING/HEMORRHAGE ★

PATHOPHYSIOLOGY

Abnormal uterine bleeding (AUB) is any bleeding from the uterus that is abnormal in volume or timing. This includes menses that occur irregularly, last for an abnormal number of days, or produce excessive blood loss. It occurs most often in adolescents and people approaching menopause. Common underlying causes of bleeding can be remembered with the mnemonic PALM-COEIN:

- **P**olyp
- **A**denomyosis
- **L**eiomyoma (fibroids)
- **M**alignancy
- **C**oagulopathy
- **O**vulatory disorder
- **E**ndometrial
- **I**atrogenic (e.g., IUD insertion)
- **N**ot otherwise classified

HELPFUL HINT
Endometriosis is a condition caused by the growth of endometrial tissue outside the uterus. It presents with intense pelvic pain, urinary symptoms, and menstrual irregularities.

DIAGNOSIS

- metrorrhagia
- menorrhagia (soaking more than 1 pad or tampon per hour or greater than 30 cc volume measured via menstrual cup)

TREATMENT AND MANAGEMENT

- control bleeding
- fluids or blood products as needed
- nonemergent presentations: referred to a gynecologist/obstetrics specialist

QUICK REVIEW QUESTION

1. A young female patient accompanied by the mother presents to the ED with a complaint of menorrhagia after experiencing amenorrhea for the past three months. What problem should the nurse anticipate when trying to obtain a truthful and complete history from the patient?

FOREIGN BODIES IN THE GYNECOLOGICAL SYSTEM

PATHOPHYSIOLOGY

FOREIGN OBJECTS in the vagina can occur in all age groups. Young children exploring their bodies may insert small objects such as crayons or marker lids. Adults may also experience forgotten tampons or have pieces of condoms left behind after sexual activity. Foreign objects may be inserted vaginally for sexual stimulation that cannot subsequently be removed, including sex toys, beads, or marbles. Objects not designed for vaginal use may lead to infection, and objects with batteries may result in chemical burns.

DIAGNOSIS

- vaginal pain, bleeding, or discharge
- abdominal or pelvic pain
- swelling of the vagina or vulva
- dysuria
- dyspareunia
- visualization of foreign body during exam
- X-ray or ultrasound showing presence of foreign body

TREATMENT AND MANAGEMENT

- analgesics
- remove object
  - □ speculum and forceps
  - □ warm water lavage of the vagina

□ sedation and/or anesthesia required for objects that cannot be removed without causing pain

QUICK REVIEW QUESTION

2. A 13-year-old female patient presents to the ED with complaints of foul-smelling, yellow-brown vaginal discharge and itching. The girl's mother reports that the girl recently started menstruating and using feminine hygiene products. What should the nurse suspect has caused these signs and symptoms?

INFECTION ★

- **CHLAMYDIA** is an STI caused by the bacteria *Chlamydia trachomatis*; left untreated, it can lead to PID, infertility, and ectopic pregnancy in women.
    □ Diagnosis: often asymptomatic, especially for men; discharge from site of infection; vaginal bleeding; dysuria; pruritus; NAAT performed on urine or swab
    □ Management: antibiotics (azithromycin [Zithromax], doxycycline); supportive treatment for symptoms

- **GENITAL HERPES** is an STI caused by the two strains of the herpes simplex virus (HSV-1 and HSV-2). The first outbreak after the initial infection is the most severe; recurrent outbreaks, which vary in frequency and duration, will generally be less severe.
    □ Diagnosis: prodrome of itching, burning, or tingling at infection site; vesicles on genitalia, perineum, or buttocks; fever, adenopathy during initial infection; PCR on swab of open lesion
    □ Management: antivirals; supportive treatment for symptoms

- **GONORRHEA** is an STI caused by the gram-negative diplococcus Neisseria gonorrhoeae; left untreated, it can lead to PID, infertility, and ectopic pregnancy.
    □ Diagnosis: usually asymptomatic; discharge from site of infection; dysuria; metrorrhagia; oropharyngeal erythema; culture or NAAT of swab
    □ Management: antibiotics (not fluoroquinolones); supportive treatment for symptoms

- **PELVIC INFLAMMATORY DISEASE (PID) IS** an infection of the upper organs of the female reproductive system, usually caused by a STI.
    □ Diagnosis: cervical, uterine, or adnexal tenderness; vaginal discharge; abdominal or low back pain; right scapular pain (Fitz-Hugh–Curtis syndrome); postcoital bleeding; metrorrhagia; dyspareunia; pleuritic URQ pain; nausea and vomiting; fever; labs show infection
    □ Management: antibiotics; supportive treatment for symptoms

- **SYPHILIS** is an STI caused by the bacteria *Treponema pallidum*. The infection progresses through four stages: primary (3 – 90 days after infection), secondary (4 – 10 weeks after infection), latent (3 months – 3 years after infection), and tertiary (> 3 years after infection).

- ☐ Signs and Symptoms (primary stage): firm, round, and painless chancres lasting 3 – 6 weeks
- ☐ Signs and Symptoms (secondary stage): rough, red rash on torso, hands, soles of feet; fever; lesions on mucous membranes; arthritis
- ☐ Signs and Symptoms (latent stage): asymptomatic
- ☐ Signs and Symptoms (tertiary stage): varies by affected system
- ☐ Diagnosis: positive VDRL, RPR, or specific treponemal antibody test
- ☐ Management: antibiotics; supportive treatment for symptoms

- ■ **Vulvovaginitis** is inflammation of the vulva and vagina. It is usually the result of an infection by bacteria, yeast, or trichomoniasis (a protozoan parasite).
  - ☐ Signs and Symptoms (general): dyspareunia, dysuria, vulvovaginal pruritis
  - ☐ Signs and Symptoms (bacterial vaginosis): malodorous white-grey vaginal discharge
  - ☐ Signs and Symptoms (vulvovaginal candidiasis): thick, white vaginal discharge with no odor (often described as "cottage cheese" like)
  - ☐ Signs and Symptoms (trichomoniasis): frothy, green-yellow vaginal discharge; vaginal inflammation ("strawberry cervix")
  - ☐ Diagnosis: culture or wet mount
  - ☐ Management: antibiotic, antifungal, or antiprotozoal as indicated

Quick Review Question

3. A 22-year-old female patient presents to the ED with white, foul-smelling vaginal discharge but no itching or urinary symptoms. What medication will the patient most likely require?

OVARIAN CYST

Pathophysiology

Ovarian cysts form in the ovaries, usually a result of an unreleased egg (follicular cyst) or failure of the corpus luteum to break down (corpus luteum cyst). Ovarian cysts are usually asymptomatic and are often found during assessments related to other conditions. However, the cysts can burst, causing intense pain; they can also increase the risk of ovarian torsion.

Diagnosis

- ■ often asymptomatic
- ■ pelvic pain, feeling of fullness, or discomfort
- ■ dyspareunia
- ■ irregular menstrual cycle

DID YOU KNOW?
Risk factors for ovarian cysts include endometriosis, infertility treatment, hormonal imbalances, hypothyroidism, tubal ligation, and PID.

- rupture: sudden, severe, unilateral pelvic pain
- transvaginal ultrasound to diagnose

TREATMENT AND MANAGEMENT

- analgesics
- fluids or blood products (for severe hemorrhage)
- surgical intervention in rare cases of continued bleeding or large cyst

QUICK REVIEW QUESTION

4. A patient arrives at the ED with vaginal bleeding and pain on the right side of the abdomen. The pregnancy test is negative, and the nurse suspects an ovarian cyst. What method definitively diagnoses an ovarian cyst?

SEXUAL ASSAULT AND BATTERY

SEXUAL ASSAULT is any unwanted sexual or physical contact or behavior that occurs without the explicit consent of the recipient. Victims of sexual assault can be male or female, adult or pediatric. It is a significantly underreported crime, and many victims know the assailant. Any patient presenting with a report of sexual assault should be treated with respect and dignity.

TREATMENT AND MANAGEMENT

- Assess for serious or emergent conditions that may require immediate treatment.
- For female patients, take a complete OB/GYN history.
- The physician or a certified sexual assault nurse examiner (SANE) may perform a sexual assault medical forensic exam (also called a sexual assault forensic exam or "rape kit") to document injuries and collect evidence.
- Follow hospital protocols for STI screening (some hospitals require it while others do not).
- All patients reporting sexual assault should be offered postexposure prophylaxis.
  - □ emergency contraception (after negative hCG test)
  - □ antibiotics and antiprotozoals (ceftriaxone, metronidazole, azithromycin and/or doxycycline)
  - □ HIV postexposure prophylaxis (PEP)
  - □ HPV vaccine
- Provide emotional support to patient.
- Provide patient with access to available resources for survivors of sexual assault, including hospital counselors and community sexual assault centers.

- Nurses should keep in mind that patients' medical records are legal documents that may be used in criminal or civil court proceedings.

- All interactions with patients should be carefully documented.

- Nurses who are asked to testify in court should confer with the hospital's legal team.

QUICK REVIEW QUESTION

5. A patient arrives at the ED stating they have been beaten and sexually assaulted. What is the nurse's priority?

GYNECOLOGICAL TRAUMA

PATHOPHYSIOLOGY

Female patients presenting with complaints of genital pain or bleeding should undergo a thorough history and physical examination. External trauma can usually be identified easily; however, internal examination will be required to evaluate for deeper injury. Vulvar injuries may include lacerations and hematomas, while vaginal trauma may present with lacerations. Uterine and cervical injuries are generally associated with pregnancy; however, they can also be caused by vaginal or abdominal trauma. Undiagnosed vaginal trauma may result in secondary issues including dyspareunia, pelvis abscesses, and fistula formations.

HELPFUL HINT

Patients may not be forthcoming with the details of gynecological trauma because of fear or embarrassment. The possibility of sexual assault or physical abuse must be considered and should be handled according to the appropriate protocols.

SIGNS AND SYMPTOMS

- pain (vaginal, external, or visceral)
- vaginal bleeding
- external laceration, ecchymosis, or mutilation
- hematuria or dysuria
- foul-smelling vaginal discharge
- labial edema
- visible wound, penetration injury, or embedded object

TREATMENT AND MANAGEMENT

- pain management
    - analgesics
    - cold compresses
- sutures for lacerations
- remove foreign object(s)

6. A 22-year-old female patient seeks treatment in the ED after falling onto a metal hurdle during a track sporting event. In triage, the patient denies vaginal bleeding but complains of throbbing pain "down there." What interventions should the nurse initiate?

ANSWER KEY

1. A young female patient may not disclose a history of sexual activity or potential pregnancy in the presence of a parent. The nurse should create an opportunity to ask these questions in a private setting such as a bathroom or exam room.

2. The start of menses can be challenging for young women. The patient may have accidently left a tampon in her vagina, which after a few weeks would cause the reported signs and symptoms.

3. A white, foul-smelling vaginal discharge with no other signs or symptoms is characteristic of bacterial vaginosis. The patient will likely be treated with a course of antibiotics such as metronidazole or clindamycin.

4. Ultrasound of the ovaries, usually transvaginal, is used to determine if there is an ovarian cyst and the status of the cyst (e.g., intact, ruptured, etc.).

5. The nurse's priority is to assess the patient for serious or life-threatening injuries. Further interventions, including forensic exams and prophylaxis, will be provided based on the patient's wishes.

6. The patient likely sustained a straddle injury and is experiencing soft tissue swelling of the labia and external genitalia. A urine sample should be obtained and the patient prepped for a manual pelvic exam. Cold compresses can be provided to decrease swelling and provide localized pain relief.

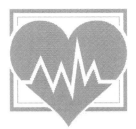

7

OBSTETRICAL EMERGENCIES

BCEN CONTENT OUTLINE

PLACENTAL DISORDERS

PATHOPHYSIOLOGY

ABRUPTIO PLACENTAE (placental abruption) occurs when the placenta separates from the uterus after the twentieth week of gestation but before delivery. Abruption can lead to life-threatening conditions, including hemorrhage and DIC. Blood loss due to abruption can be difficult to quantify as blood may accumulate behind the placenta (CONCEALED ABRUPTION) rather than exiting through the vagina.

DID YOU KNOW?

Risk factors for abruptio placentae include hypertension, preeclampsia, blunt trauma, smoking, and cocaine use.

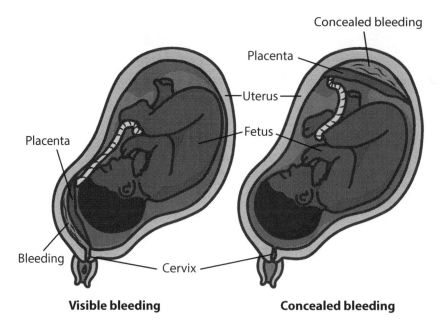

Figure 7.1. Abruptio Placentae

PLACENTA PREVIA occurs when the placenta partially or completely covers the internal orifice of the cervix. A low lying placenta is located ≤ 2 cm from the cervix but does not cover it. Placenta previa is usually asymptomatic and is found on routine prenatal ultrasounds. The presence of previa makes the placenta susceptible to rupture or hemorrhage and necessitates a cesarean delivery.

Placenta previa is correlated with **PLACENTA ACCRETA**, particularly in women who have had multiple previous cesarean deliveries. In placenta accreta, the placenta attaches abnormally deeply into the myometrium. Because the placenta cannot detach from the uterus after delivery, placenta accreta can lead to hemorrhage and requires a hysterectomy.

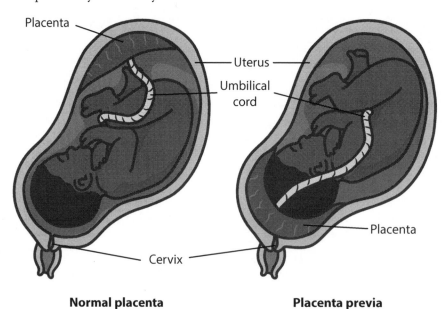

Figure 7.2. Placenta Previa

Table 7.1. Diagnosis of Abruptio Placentae and Placenta Previa

	ABRUPTIO PLACENTAE	PLACENTA PREVIA
ONSET OF SYMPTOMS	sudden and intense bleeding with pain	asymptomatic or painless bleeding
BLEEDING	bleeding may be vaginal or concealed	vaginal bleeding
UTERINE TONE	firm	soft and relaxed
IMAGING	transabdominal or transvaginal ultrasound	transabdominal or transvaginal ultrasound; no rectal or cervical exam until placenta placement is known

TREATMENT AND MANAGEMENT

- fetal heart rate monitoring
- monitor mother for signs of hemodynamic instability
- RhoGAM if mother is Rh negative
- IV fluids or blood products as needed
- patient admitted stat to OB

QUICK REVIEW QUESTION

1. What signs or symptoms indicate a significant separation of the placenta from the uterus?

ECTOPIC PREGNANCY

PATHOPHYSIOLOGY

In an **ECTOPIC PREGNANCY**, the blastocyst implants in a location other than the uterus. In > 95% of cases, implantation occurs in the fallopian tubes (tubal pregnancy), but implantation can also occur in the ovaries, cervix, or abdominal cavity. Ectopic pregnancies are most often caused by tubal irregularities that are congenital or the result of infection or surgery. A tubal pregnancy may rupture the fallopian tube, causing a life-threatening hemorrhage.

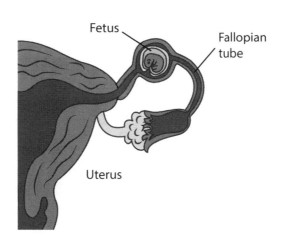

Figure 7.3. Ectopic Pregnancy (Tubal Pregnancy)

DIAGNOSIS

- may be asymptomatic
- vaginal bleeding
- lower abdominal pain
- s/s of hemorrhage
- pregnancy confirmation with urine or serum hCG
- transvaginal ultrasound to locate pregnancy

TREATMENT AND MANAGEMENT

- RhoGAM if mother is Rh negative
- hemodynamically unstable patients: stabilize and prepare for surgery
- hemodynamically stable patients: OB referral for surgery or treatment with methotrexate

QUICK REVIEW QUESTION

2. A sexually active 19-year-old presents to the ED with vaginal bleeding and intermittent LLQ abdominal pain. Vital signs are stable, abdomen is tender, and the patient's uterus is soft and slightly enlarged. An ultrasound assessment confirms an ectopic pregnancy. What will be the most likely intervention for this patient?

★ LABOR AND DELIVERY

PATHOPHYSIOLOGY

Labor and delivery occurs in 3 stages.

- Stage 1: onset of labor to full cervical dilation (12 – 16 hours)
- Stage 2: cervical dilation to expulsion of fetus (2 – 3 hours)
- Stage 3: delivery of placenta (10 – 12 minutes)

HELPFUL HINT

Umbilical cord prolapse occurs when the cord presents alongside (occult) or ahead of (overt) the presenting fetus during delivery. Exposure of the cord makes it vulnerable to compression or rupture, which disrupts blood flow to the fetus.

Delivery is IMMINENT if the fetus is visible and/or the mother reports the urge to push with contractions. Alternatively, delivery can be considered imminent if the cervix is fully dilated (10 cm) and contractions are < 2 minutes apart.

Contractions and cervical dilation before the thirty-seventh week of gestation is PRETERM LABOR. If preterm labor begins between 34 and 37 weeks with no other complications, the patient should be transferred to the labor and delivery setting if delivery is not imminent. When preterm labor begins at < 34 weeks, the mother should be transferred to OB for treatment to delay delivery.

DIAGNOSIS

- ruptured amniotic membrane ("water broke")
- dilation of cervix
- contractions

- urge to push
- pelvic exam: assess cervical dilation
- fetal Doppler to assess fetal heart rate
- transabdominal ultrasound: to identify presentation and number of fetus(es) and assess for possible complications

TREATMENT AND MANAGEMENT

- Assess patient to determine stage of labor and gestational age.
  - □ preterm labor or complications: OB consult stat
  - □ delivery not imminent: patient should be transferred to OB for delivery
  - □ delivery imminent and no complications: delivery will take place in the ED
- Monitor maternal blood pressure, heart rate, and contractions.
- Monitor fetal heart rate.
- Administer RhoGAM if mother is Rh negative.
- Administer betamethasone for imminent delivery of fetus < 34 weeks.
- Position mother is lithotomy position for delivery.
- Clean perineum with antiseptic.
- Care of newborn postdelivery:
  - □ Wipe nose and mouth; suction airway if obstructed.
  - □ Dry and stimulate newborn.
  - □ Assign Apgar score.
- Care of mother postdelivery:
  - □ Deliver placenta.
  - □ Administer oxytocin IM or perform fundal massage.
  - □ Monitor for signs of hemorrhage.

HELPFUL HINT
Apgar scoring is 0 to 2 points for:
- neonatal heart rate
- respiratory effort
- muscle tone
- reflex irritability
- color

QUICK REVIEW QUESTION

3. A 25-year-old full-term patient presents to the ED stating her water broke and that she is in labor. A quick assessment reveals the cervix is fully dilated and the head is crowning. What is the nurse's priority?

POSTPARTUM HEMORRHAGE ★

PATHOPHYSIOLOGY

POSTPARTUM HEMORRHAGE is bleeding that occurs any time after delivery up to 12 weeks postpartum and exceeds 1000 ml or that causes symptoms of hypovolemia. Primary hemorrhage occurs during the first 24 hours after delivery; secondary hemorrhage occurs between 24 hours and 12 weeks postpartum. The etiology of hemorrhage varies.

- trauma: lacerations to uterus or vagina
- uterine atony: failure of the uterus to contract after delivery, often because of placental disorders
- retained tissue
- coagulation disorders
- subinvolution of the placental site: persistence of dilated arteries in placenta or uterus postpartum
- infection

DIAGNOSIS

- vaginal bleeding
- s/s of hypovolemia

TREATMENT AND MANAGEMENT

- IV fluids and blood products as needed
- tranexamic acid (to promote clotting)
- prep for surgery

QUICK REVIEW QUESTION

4. A patient presents to the ED with heavy vaginal bleeding after a home birth. Her blood pressure is 110/65 mm Hg, her HR is 118, and her RR is 24. What interventions should the nurse prepare for?

HYPEREMESIS GRAVIDARUM

PATHOPHYSIOLOGY

HYPEREMESIS GRAVIDARUM is severe nausea and vomiting that occurs during pregnancy. While there is no definitive diagnostic line between hyperemesis and common "morning sickness," hyperemesis is generally defined as frequent vomiting that results in weight loss and ketonuria. Severe vomiting can lead to dehydration, hypovolemia, and electrolyte imbalances. Hyperemesis usually presents around 6 weeks gestation and resolves around 16 to 20 weeks. However, for some women it may persist until delivery.

DIAGNOSIS

- persistent vomiting (> 3 times per day)
- weight loss of > 5 pounds or > 5% of body weight
- s/s of hypovolemia

TREATMENT AND MANAGEMENT

- IV fluids
  - ☐ initial infusion of lactated Ringer's followed by dextrose
  - ☐ urine output 100 ml/hour

- replace lost vitamins and minerals: IV thiamine, IV multivitamin, IV magnesium, calcium, or phosphorus as indicated by labs
- antiemetics

QUICK REVIEW QUESTION

5. How is hyperemesis gravidarum differentiated from morning sickness?

NEONATAL RESUSCITATION

PATHOPHYSIOLOGY

The transition to extrauterine life requires a complex series of changes in the cardiopulmonary system of a neonate. The alveoli in the neonate's lungs expand, usually beginning with the first breath, and the lungs are cleared of fluid. In addition, the clamping of the umbilical cord combined with the expansion of the lungs raises the neonate's blood pressure and pushes blood into the vasculature of the lungs.

A small number of neonates (around 10%) will require intervention to establish ventilation. Poor respiratory performance can have a number of causes:

- blocked airway
- lack of respiratory effort (usually the result of musculature or neurological deficits)
- persistent pulmonary hypertension in the newborn
- heart or lung defects
- preterm labor (lungs are not mature enough to clear and expand)

DIAGNOSIS

- absence of spontaneous breath
- absence of vigorous cry
- airway obstruction (nares and/or trachea)
- cyanosis
- poor muscle tone

RESUSCITATION PROCEDURES

- Stimulate the neonate by rubbing back, feet, and/or chest vigorously.
- Prevent heat loss by placing child in warmer.
- Clear airway of obstructions using bulb suction or wall suction (low suction).
- If stimulation and warming do not work, activate neonatal resuscitation code.
- Neonatal resuscitation is a specialized skill and requires supplemental education and certification.

- The ED nurse should be prepared to provide basic resuscitation of a neonate until the appropriate caregivers can arrive.
- Apply oxygen with positive pressure ventilation.
- If the neonate is apneic and the heart rate is < 60, initiate CPR.

QUICK REVIEW QUESTION

6. A neonate delivered in the ED is receiving resuscitation measures. What assessment criteria would indicate that resuscitation measures have been successful?

POSTPARTUM INFECTION

PATHOPHYSIOLOGY

Postpartum patients are frequently discharged soon after delivery and may develop POSTPARTUM INFECTIONS at home that require further treatment. Possible sites of infection include the endometrium (ENDOMETRITIS), surgical incisions, breasts (mastitis), and urinary tract. The infection may spread and lead to septicemia, peritonitis, or sepsis. Endometritis is the most common postpartum infection.

DIAGNOSIS

- fever of ≥ 100.4°F (38°C):
  - □ on more than 2 of the first 10 days postpartum
  - □ maintained over 24 hours after the end of the first day postpartum
- endometritis: uterine tenderness, midline lower abdominal pain
- surgical incision infection: erythema and inflammation at incision, purulent exudate
- mastitis: erythema and tenderness in breast
- labs show infection

TREATMENT AND MANAGEMENT

- endometritis and UTI: antibiotics, analgesics, antipyretics
- surgical incision: drain, irrigate, and debride wound
- mastitis: antibiotics, analgesics, antipyretics, empty breast of milk

HELPFUL HINT
Antibiotics are not usually prescribed for surgical incision infections.

QUICK REVIEW QUESTION

7. A postpartum patient returns to the ED 4 days following discharge from an uncomplicated vaginal delivery. She has a temperature of 101°F (38.3°C) and assessment shows erythema and discharge with an odor at her episiotomy site. What interventions should the nurse anticipate?

PREECLAMPSIA AND ECLAMPSIA ★

PATHOPHYSIOLOGY

PREECLAMPSIA is a syndrome caused by abnormalities in the placental vasculature. The syndrome is characterized by hypertension in the mother paired with either proteinuria or end-organ dysfunction. Symptoms can appear after the twentieth week of pregnancy and most commonly appear after 34 weeks. In most cases, preeclampsia will resolve after delivery, but symptoms can develop up to 4 weeks postpartum. Because preeclampsia is usually diagnosed during routine prenatal care, postpartum preeclampsia most commonly presents in the ED.

Preeclampsia is classified as being either with or without severe features. Preeclampsia with severe features can lead to life-threatening complications, including eclampsia, pulmonary edema, and abruptio placentae.

ECLAMPSIA is the onset of tonic-clonic seizures in women with preeclampsia. Eclampsia can occur ante-, intra-, or postpartum. It is an emergent condition that requires immediate medical intervention.

DIAGNOSIS

- hypertension: systolic BP > 140 mmHg or diastolic BP > 90 mmHg
- facial edema
- rapid weight gain (> 5 pounds a week)
- severe preeclampsia: headache, epigastric pain, pitting edema
- eclampsia: tonic-clonic seizures
- proteinuria diagnosed through urine sample:
  - □ 24-hour urine protein: ≥ 0.3 g
  - □ urine dipstick protein: ≥ 1+ (mild preeclampsia) to ≥ 3+ (severe preeclampsia)
  - □ serum creatinine: > 1.2 mg/dL indicates severe preeclampsia

TREATMENT AND MANAGEMENT

- antihypertensives (labetalol, hydralazine, or short-acting nifedipine)
- prophylactic magnesium (to prevent seizures)
- admit to OB

QUICK REVIEW QUESTION

8. A patient who is 37 weeks pregnant presents to the ED. Assessment finds BP 162/112, P 88, R 24, reflexes +3/+4, and her urine tests positive for ketones. What intervention should the nurse be prepared for?

HELLP SYNDROME

PATHOPHYSIOLOGY

HELLP SYNDROME is currently believed to be a form of preeclampsia, although the relationship between the two disorders is controversial and not well understood. Around 85% of women diagnosed with HELLP will also present with symptoms of preeclampsia (hypertension and proteinuria). HELLP is characterized by:

- hemolysis (H)
- elevated liver enzymes (EL)
- low platelet count (LP)

DIAGNOSIS

- hypertension: systolic > 140 mmHg or diastolic > 90 mmHg
- RUQ abdominal pain
- nausea and vomiting
- severe headache or visual disturbances
- urine protein consistent with preeclampsia diagnosis
- schistocytes on blood smear
- platelets: ≤ 100,000 cells/μL
- total bilirubin: ≥ 1.2 mg/dL
- AST: > 70 units/L

TREATMENT AND MANAGEMENT

- antihypertensives (labetalol, hydralazine, or short-acting nifedipine)
- prophylactic magnesium (to prevent seizures)
- admit to OB

QUICK REVIEW QUESTION

9. What abnormal laboratory values confirm the diagnosis of HELLP?

SPONTANEOUS ABORTION

PATHOPHYSIOLOGY

SPONTANEOUS ABORTION (miscarriage) is the loss of a pregnancy before the twentieth week of gestation. (Death of the fetus after the twentieth week is commonly referred to as a **STILLBIRTH.**) Spontaneous abortions are a common complication of early pregnancy. They can occur because of chromosomal or congenital abnormalities, material infection or disorders, or trauma.

Spontaneous abortions are classified by the location of the embryo/fetus and cervical dilation.

- **MISSED ABORTION**: occurs when the embryo/fetus is nonviable but has not been passed from the uterus and the cervix is closed

- **THREATENED ABORTION**: occurs when the patient has vaginal bleeding before 20 weeks and the cervix is closed; may progress to incomplete or complete abortion

- **INEVITABLE ABORTION**: occurs when the patient has vaginal bleeding and the cervix is dilated but the embryo/fetus remains in the uterus; often accompanied by abdominal pain or cramps

- **INCOMPLETE ABORTION**: occurs when the patient has vaginal bleeding, the cervix is dilated, and the embryo/fetus is found in the cervical canal

- **COMPLETE ABORTION**: occurs when the embryo/fetus has been completely expelled from the uterus and cervix and the cervix is closed

- **SEPTIC ABORTION**: occurs when the abortion is accompanied by uterine infection; it is a life-threatening condition that requires immediate medical intervention

DIAGNOSIS

- vaginal bleeding
- passage of fetal tissue
- radiating pelvic pain
- signs and symptoms of cessation of pregnancy (e.g., nausea, breast tenderness)
- s/s of infection with septic abortion
- fetal Doppler to assess for fetal cardiac activity
- transvaginal ultrasound to confirm pregnancy loss

TREATMENT AND MANAGEMENT

- RhoGAM if mother is Rh negative
- analgesics
- monitor patient for hemodynamic instability
- OB referral
- septic abortion: antibiotics and prep patient for surgery

QUICK REVIEW QUESTION

10. A patient in the first trimester is admitted to the ED with complaints of abdominal cramping and spotting over the last 18 hours. During the assessment the nurse is palpating the breast for tenderness and the patient states that the tenderness is gone. Why is the lack of tenderness to the breast a concern for the nurse?

OBSTETRICAL TRAUMA

PATHOPHYSIOLOGY

Trauma is the leading nonobstetric cause of death for pregnant people. Common causes of trauma include MVAs, falls, and intimate partner violence. Trauma is categorized as major if it involves the abdomen, includes high force, or results in vaginal bleeding or decreased fetal movement. Minor trauma does not involve the abdomen and may include no obvious signs and symptoms. However, minor trauma can still be fatal for mother or fetus, so a thorough assessment should be done on any trauma patient who may be pregnant.

In the ED, the patient should be assessed and stabilized before the fetus is assessed. Pregnant patients presenting to the ED should be evaluated for any non–pregnancy-related issues and then referred to OB if necessary.

DIAGNOSIS

- visible signs and symptoms of injury, including ecchymosis and lacerations
- vaginal bleeding
- tense abdomen
- decreased uterine tone
- presence of amniotic fluid due to membrane rupture
- transvaginal ultrasound to assess fetus, locate placenta, and assess for abruption
- FAST ultrasound to assess for hemorrhage if suspected

TREATMENT AND MANAGEMENT

- priority: assess mother's ABCs
- oxygen, respiratory intervention, or cardiac resuscitation as needed
- IV fluids or blood products as needed
- RhoGAM if mother is Rh negative
- betamethasone for imminent delivery of fetus < 34 weeks
- monitor fetal HR and uterine contractions
- OB consult for all obstetric trauma patients

HELPFUL HINT

Betamethasone is a corticosteroid that speeds up fetal lung development. It is administered to the mother if there is a high risk of preterm labor (< 34 weeks).

QUICK REVIEW QUESTION

11. A patient in the third trimester is admitted to the ED after a fall. The assessment shows no vaginal bleeding, but the patient's H/H is low. What should the nurse suspect?

ANSWER KEY

1. Significant separation of the placenta results in hemorrhage and rapid blood loss. Patients will show signs of hypovolemia, including heavy vaginal bleeding (unless abruption is concealed), hypotension, tachycardia, tachypnea, reduced urine output, and abnormal fetal heart rate.

2. Because the patient is stable, refer to OB for assessment. The pregnancy will most likely be terminated using methotrexate or surgically.

3. The nurse should prepare the patient for delivery. Obtain maternal vital signs and fetal heart rate. Place the mother in the lithotomy position and raise the head of the bed. Clean the perineum with antiseptic. Continue to check fetal heart rate and be prepared to aid with delivery of newborn.

4. The patient is showing early signs of hypovolemia (tachycardia and tachypnea accompanied by heavy blood loss). The nurse should monitor the patient for signs of hemodynamic instability and be prepared to deliver fluids or blood products as necessary. Once stable, the patient should be prepared for surgery.

5. Morning sickness is the common term for mild nausea and vomiting during early pregnancy. It does not usually affect fluid levels and can be managed with lifestyle changes. Hyperemesis gravidarum is defined as persistent nausea and vomiting in early pregnancy that leads to weight loss (> 5 pounds), dehydration, and possible hypovolemia and electrolyte imbalances.

6. The goal of resuscitation is for the neonate to have spontaneous respiration and a heart rate ≥ 100 bpm. The neonate's oxygen saturation should also be monitored and should reach 85% to 95% by 10 minutes postdelivery.

7. The patient most likely has a postpartum infection at the episiotomy site. The nurse should be prepared to drain and clean the wound and provide treatment for pain (ice packs or NSAIDs). The nurse may also be asked to order a culture and sensitivity of the discharge and administer broad-spectrum antibiotics.

8. The patient is presenting with signs and symptoms of preeclampsia. The nurse should be prepared to administer antihypertensives and magnesium and to begin maternal and fetal monitoring.

9. Hemolysis (H), elevated liver enzymes (EL), and a low platelet count (LP).

10. A loss or lack of tenderness indicates hormone levels have decreased and a spontaneous abortion is in progress or is imminent.

11. The nurse should suspect occult bleeding. The patient will require an ultrasound to assess for an abruption or other sources of bleeding, and may need blood products. This patient will likely be admitted to OB.

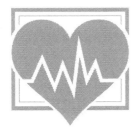

8

PSYCHOSOCIAL EMERGENCIES

BCEN CONTENT OUTLINE

✱ **A. ABUSE AND NEGLECT**

✱ **B. AGGRESSIVE/VIOLENT BEHAVIOR**

   C. Anxiety/panic

   D. Bipolar disorder

   E. Depression

   F. Homicidal ideation

   G. Psychosis

   H. Situational crisis (e.g., job loss, relationship issues, unexpected death)

✱ **I. SUICIDAL IDEATION**

ABUSE AND NEGLECT ✱

CHARACTERISTICS

Patients presenting in the ED with concern for **ABUSE** and **NEGLECT** generally fall into one of three categories: domestic abuse, child abuse/neglect, and geriatric abuse/neglect. Nursing assessment for each of these concerns begins at triage, and every patient presenting to the ED should be screened for signs or indications of neglect. Abuse can include both physical and emotional abuse; neglect may be on the part of caregivers or self.

DIAGNOSIS

- physical s/s: unexplained injuries, fractures or bruising at different stages of healing, poor hygiene, weight loss or gain
- emotional s/s: severe mood swings or changes, agitation, depression, suicidal ideation

TREATMENT AND MANAGEMENT

- Protected populations (including pediatric and geriatric patients) require obligatory reporting of suspected abuse and neglect.

- The priority treatment of the abused or neglected patient should focus on physical injuries.

- Consideration should be made for emotional needs that result from abuse and neglect.
  - ☐ Provide same-gender caregivers or a same-gender chaperone for exams.
  - ☐ Use organizational resources to provide support for the patient.
  - ☐ Ask permission to touch the patient or narrate the physical exam.
  - ☐ Warn the patient when and where they will be touched during the exam.

QUICK REVIEW QUESTION

1. A male pediatric patient arrives at the ED with a chief complaint of abdominal pain. Upon assessment, the nurse discovers bruising to the abdomen, back, and arms that appears to be in different stages of healing. The mother of the patient is at the bedside. What is the nurse's next action?

★ AGGRESSIVE OR VIOLENT BEHAVIOR

CHARACTERISTICS

Aggressive or violent behavior in patients may occur for many reasons, including:

- crisis or psychosis
- altered mental status
- influence of drugs or alcohol
- underlying organic processes
- traumatic brain injuries
- urosepsis, especially in patients > 65
- acute dementia or Alzheimer's disease

TREATMENT AND MANAGEMENT

- Management ranges from verbal de-escalation to mechanical restraint of the violent patient.

- De-escalation strategies:
  - ☐ verbal redirection
  - ☐ allowing the patient to express needs
  - ☐ allowing the patient to exercise
  - ☐ decreased environmental stimulation (quiet room time)
  - ☐ PRN medication administration (as requested by patient)

- Restraints may be used.
  - □ should be used conservatively
  - □ only for patients whose behavior cannot be controlled through less restrictive measures
  - □ require frequent assessment (every 5 – 15 minutes depending on organizational policy)
  - □ check vitals, assess pain, assess circulation and skin integrity of all restrained extremities, and address restroom needs
  - □ should be removed as soon as they are deemed unnecessary for patient and staff safety
- In patients with acute agitation, medications can be administered: olanzapine (Zyprexa), haloperidol (Haldol), or risperidone (Risperdal)

QUICK REVIEW QUESTION

2. A patient was placed in mechanical restraints after demonstrating violent and aggressive behavior toward nursing staff. It has been 15 minutes since the restraints were applied, and the nurse is preparing to assess the patient. What will the nurse include in her assessment?

ANXIETY AND PANIC

CHARACTERISTICS

ANXIETY is feelings of fear, apprehension, and worry that can be characterized as mild, moderate, or severe (panic). Anxiety will impact other functions such as the respiratory, cardiac, and gastrointestinal systems. A key nursing consideration is to assess for organic causes for reported symptoms, as other life-threatening illnesses may present with similar symptoms.

DIAGNOSIS

- sudden onset of fear, worry, concern
- physical manifestations: palpitations or chest pain, dyspnea, diaphoresis, nausea

TREATMENT AND MANAGEMENT

- Treatment of anxiety should be targeted at the level of anxiety the patient presents with (mild to panic).
- Non-pharmacological interventions include:
  - □ Place patient in calm environment.
  - □ Encourage rhythmic breathing.
  - □ Offer social support if possible.
- Pharmacological interventions (fast-acting anxiolytics) include:
  - □ benzodiazepines (diazepam [Valium], lorazepam [Ativan])
  - □ antihistamines (hydroxyzine)

3. A patient presents to the ED stating he was in a movie theater and suddenly began to feel fearful, apprehensive, and on edge. He is feeling mild chest pain and shortness of breath. What should the nurse ask in the assessment of this patient?

BIPOLAR DISORDER

CHARACTERISTICS

BIPOLAR DISORDER (also known as manic-depressive illness) is characterized by shifts in mood accompanied by changes in activity and energy. These shifts are categorized as manic behaviors or depressive behaviors. Severe episodes of either mania or depression can also result in psychosis, characterized by hallucinations or delusions.

DIAGNOSIS

- manic behavior: feelings of elation, high levels of energy, difficulty sleeping, engaging in high-risk activities
- depressive behavior: deep or intense feelings of sadness, decreased energy levels, sleep disturbances, suicidal ideation or focus on death

TREATMENT AND MANAGEMENT

- Treatment in ED addresses the exacerbations of the disorder (i.e., patients "in crisis").
- Assess for and treat conditions related to manic or depressive behaviors (e.g., dehydration, trauma injuries).
- Extreme or long-term mania requires immediate hospitalization and medical attention.
- Medications may be used to treat symptoms of exacerbations.
  - □ mood stabilizers (lithium, lamotrigine [Lamictal])
  - □ atypical antipsychotics (risperidone, aripiprazole [Abilify])
  - □ antipsychotics and antidepressants (olanzapine, quetiapine [Seroquel])

QUICK REVIEW QUESTION

4. What are some key considerations in the assessment of a patient with bipolar disorder on the third day of a manic episode?

DEPRESSION AND DYSTHYMIC DISORDER

CHARACTERISTICS

DEPRESSION is a mood disorder that has both emotional and physical symptoms. Patients who are depressed report feelings of sadness and hopelessness that last longer than two weeks, and they often will report feelings of suicidality along with feelings of hopelessness and sadness. Depression can manifest as an exacerbation of bipolar disorder or as its own disease process.

DIAGNOSIS

- feelings of sadness or tearfulness
- irritability, increased anger, outbursts
- decreased interest in things that were once interesting
- sleep changes (too much or too little sleep)
- trouble concentrating
- increased anxiety

TREATMENT AND MANAGEMENT

- Every patient presenting to the ED should be screened for depression.
- Management of depression is long-term treatment with antidepressants and therapy.
- Symptoms associated with depression can result from an underlying illness (e.g., metabolic disorders); these should be ruled out prior to diagnosis and treatment for depression.

QUICK REVIEW QUESTION

5. A nurse is performing an assessment of a patient with a chief complaint of fatigue. The patient tells the nurse that he has felt hopeless recently and has not slept well for the last 2 or 3 weeks. What follow-up questions should the nurse ask this patient?

HOMICIDAL IDEATION
CHARACTERISTICS

HOMICIDAL IDEATION is characterized by feelings of intent to harm other people, either groups or individuals.

TREATMENT AND MANAGEMENT

- Assess for level of intent.
- If the patient identifies an individual or group, the nurse and physician should determine if they are obligated to report the threat to law enforcement or to the individual or group.

QUICK REVIEW QUESTION

6. During triage, a patient expresses to the triage nurse that he wants to kill his boss. What should the nurse do next?

HELPFUL HINT
The legal requirements for a *psychiatric emergency hold* vary by state. In most locations, patients can be involuntarily held for 48 to 72 hours if they are a danger to themselves or others.

PSYCHOSIS

CHARACTERISTICS

HELPFUL HINT

Schizophrenia is a chronic psychotic condition that is characterized by bouts of psychosis, hallucinations, and disorganized speech. Positive symptoms of schizophrenia are those not normally seen in healthy persons, and negative symptoms are disruptions of normal behaviors.

A patient experiencing an episode of **PSYCHOSIS** will have delusions, hallucinations, paranoia, suicidal or homicidal ideation, and disturbances in thinking and perceptions. Psychosis can be the result of organic illnesses or an exacerbation of an existing or new-onset mental illness such as schizophrenia or bipolar disorder.

TREATMENT AND MANAGEMENT

- Pharmacological intervention may be needed if patient is a threat to self or others.
- Assess for and treat underlying causes of psychosis.
- Psychiatric consult required with possible commitment to inpatient mental health unit.

QUICK REVIEW QUESTION

7. What are key nursing interventions for a patient in the ED presenting with acute psychosis?

SITUATIONAL CRISIS

CHARACTERISTICS

A **SITUATIONAL CRISIS** is an acute change or event in a patient's life that may lead to feelings of anxiety, fear, depression, or other mental or emotional illness concerns. Examples of a situational crisis can include:

- divorce
- rape or sexual assault
- domestic violence or abuse
- loss of a job/retirement from a job
- loss of a family member
- any event that creates crisis from a patient's perspective

Nurses should understand that the crisis is as problematic as the patient perceives it to be. The key distinction is not the nature of the event, but the patient's response to the event. Patients may self-refer for situational crises, or the ED nurse may discover that the patient is experiencing a situational crisis during the course of the ED visit.

TREATMENT AND MANAGEMENT

- Assess for patient safety and suicidal ideation.
- Provide a safe environment for the patient.
- Administer anxiolytic medications as necessary.
- Refer to the appropriate crisis resources.

8. A nurse is caring for a patient in the ED who has presented with a situational crisis. The patient has made a recent attempt at self-harm. What is the nurse's priority for this patient?

SUICIDAL IDEATION AND BEHAVIOR ★

CHARACTERISTICS

SUICIDAL IDEATION is characterized by feelings or thoughts of attempting or considering suicide. Patients exhibiting suicidal ideation may have vague thoughts without a distinct plan, or they may have a specific plan and the means to carry it out.

DIAGNOSIS

- Screen for suicidal ideation in all patients.
  - □ Ask directly if the patient is considering suicide or has recently or in the past attempted suicide.
  - □ If so, does the patient have a concrete plan to carry it out?
- Determine the presence of risk factors such as history of substance abuse or recent loss of a family member.
- Assess the presence of social supports for the patient.

TREATMENT AND MANAGEMENT

- Secure all weapons in the patient's possession.
- Secure a contract of safety with the patient. (Patient will sign a contract that states they will remain safe while in the hospital and in the future.)
- Create an environment of safety for the patient.
- Establish 1:1 watch or line-of-sight supervision for the patient.
- Assess for admission based on the severity of suicidal ideation or behavior.
- Before discharge, patient will be evaluated by psychiatrist, or ED provider will consult psychiatry.

QUICK REVIEW QUESTION

9. How can the nurse address patient and staff safety when a patient reports thoughts of self-harm?

ANSWER KEY

1. The nurse should complete the physical assessment and discuss these findings with the ED physician. She should then complete the screening for child abuse and follow local policy on mandatory reporting of suspected child abuse.

2. The nurse should assess the status of the patient, including orientation, vital signs, neurovascular status of the extremities restrained, and skin integrity at the restraint points.

3. The nurse should obtain prior medical history to include cardiac and respiratory concerns and find out if the patient has a history of anxiety reactions in the past. The nurse should be prepared to address all life-threatening illnesses before addressing anxiety.

4. The nurse should do a physical assessment to include vital signs and sleep and eating habits to determine if the patient is adequately hydrated and fed. The nurse should determine if the patient has participated in any high-risk activities that may have either long-term or acute consequences to their health.

5. The nurse should use the statements from the patient to consider organic causes for the fatigue and difficulty sleeping but should also ask further questions regarding the patient's emotional and psychological state, including those about suicidal ideation and feelings of safety.

6. The nurse should determine if the patient is in possession of any weapons and follow organizational policy regarding notifying security and the emergency physician of the patient's intent.

7. Address underlying causes of psychosis as well as resultant symptoms or injuries; request psychiatric consultation; prepare for involuntary commitment; provide a safe environment for the patient until the crisis can be addressed.

8. Providing for the patient's safety while in the ED is the nurse's priority.

9. The nurse should get a detailed accounting of the patient's plan for self-harm as well as determine if the patient is in possession of any objects or weapons that could cause harm to the patient or to the staff.

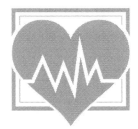

9

MEDICAL EMERGENCIES

BCEN CONTENT OUTLINE

★ **A.** **ALLERGIC REACTIONS AND ANAPHYLAXIS**

 B. Blood dyscrasias

   1. Hemophilia

   2. Other coagulopathies (e.g., anticoagulant medications, thrombocytopenia)

   3. Leukemia

   4. Sickle cell crisis

 C. Disseminated intravascular coagulation (DIC)

★ **D.** **ELECTROLYTE/FLUID IMBALANCE**

 E. Endocrine conditions

   1. Adrenal

★ **2.** **GLUCOSE RELATED CONDITIONS**

   3. Thyroid

★ **F.** **FEVER**

 G. Immunocompromise (e.g., HIV/AIDS, patients receiving chemotherapy)

 H. Renal failure

★ **I.** **SEPSIS AND SEPTIC SHOCK**

ALLERGIC REACTIONS AND ANAPHYLAXIS

Allergic Reactions

PATHOPHYSIOLOGY

An **ALLERGIC REACTION** occurs when an irritant or allergen protein enters the body by inhalation, ingestion, or topical exposure. The allergen initiates a response from the immune system, which triggers acute inflammation and vasodilation.

SIGNS AND SYMPTOMS

- topical dermatitis
- urticaria (hives)
- rhinorrhea and sneezing
- itchy skin, nose, mouth, or eyes
- circumoral tingling or pallor

TREATMENT AND MANAGEMENT

- pharmacological intervention based on location and severity of symptoms
- H1 antihistamines (diphenhydramine [Benadryl])
- PO or IV glucocorticoid (methylprednisolone, prednisone) for severe symptoms
- glucocorticoid or antihistamine nasal sprays for nasal congestion
- bronchodilator (albuterol) for respiratory symptoms
- topical antihistamines or steroids for skin symptoms

QUICK REVIEW QUESTION

1. A patient arrives at the ED with diffuse poison ivy to the lower extremities, upper extremities, chest, and neck. The patient describes having taken 50 mg of loratadine (Claritin) by mouth prior to arrival. What other medications should the nurse anticipate administering?

★ Anaphylactic Shock

PATHOPHYSIOLOGY

ANAPHYLACTIC SHOCK (OR ANAPHYLAXIS) is a life-threatening, severe allergic reaction that causes symptomatic vasodilation and bronchoconstriction. The most common causes of anaphylactic shock are food allergens, medications, and insect venom.

SIGNS AND SYMPTOMS

- respiratory distress (can be severe): dyspnea, wheezing, cough
- throat tightness and hoarseness
- dysphagia
- edema in face, lips, or tongue
- skin pallor or flushing
- hypotension
- weakness

- syncope or presyncope
- vomiting or diarrhea
- altered mental status
- sense of doom, anxiety, or confusion
- uterine contractions during pregnancy

TREATMENT AND MANAGEMENT

- first-line treatment: IM epinephrine
  - ☐ EpiPen or 1:1,000 IM 0.01 mg/kg, for a maximum dose of 0.5 mg
  - ☐ may repeat IM dose after 5 minutes
  - ☐ patients who have self-administered an EpiPen monitored for at least 4 hours
- second-line treatment
  - ☐ oxygen
  - ☐ medication for allergic reaction: H1 antihistamines bronchodilator, glucocorticoid
  - ☐ IV glucagon
  - ☐ fluid resuscitation with 0.9% normal saline bolus

HELPFUL HINT
Doses of 1:10,000 – 1:100,000 IV epinephrine are used for cardiac arrest.

QUICK REVIEW QUESTION

2. A patient from an MVC is sent to radiology for a CT scan with contrast. Upon returning, the patient complains of dyspnea and dizziness and has hoarseness. What medication should the nurse anticipate giving?

BLOOD DYSCRASIAS

Hemophilia

PATHOPHYSIOLOGY

HEMOPHILIA is a recessive, X-chromosome-linked bleeding disorder characterized by the lack of coagulation factor VIII (hemophilia A), factor IX (hemophilia B), or factor XI (hemophilia C). The deficiency in coagulation factors causes abnormal bleeding after an injury or medical procedures, and spontaneous bleeding can occur in patients with severe hemophilia. Hemophilia is usually diagnosed in infancy or childhood, but mild forms may not be diagnosed until the patient experiences injury or surgery later in life.

DID YOU KNOW?
Hemarthrosis, bleeding into the joints, is one of the most common presentations of hemophilia.

DIAGNOSIS

- excessive bleeding
- prolonged aPTT
- normal platelet count and PT
- decreased activity level for factors VIII, IX, or XI

- first line: factor VIII for hemophilia A or factor IX for hemophilia B
- standard treatment protocols for bleeding/hemorrhage

QUICK REVIEW QUESTION

3. An 8-year-old boy with a known history of hemophilia A arrives at the ED after sustaining a closed radial ulna fracture when he fell off a swing at school. What intervention should the nurse anticipate performing first?

Thrombocytopenia

- **THROMBOCYTOPENIA** is an abnormally low platelet level that can lead to severe bleeding or thrombosis. It can generally be classified by the number of platelets:
  - mild: 100,000 – 150,000/μL
  - moderate: 50,000 – 100,000/μL
  - severe: < 50,000/μL

- Thrombocytopenia has a diverse etiology. it is commonly seen in patients with cancer, bone marrow disorders, sepsis, chronic liver disease, and autoimmune diseases.

- **HEPARIN-INDUCED THROMBOCYTOPENIA (HIT)** is acute-onset thrombocytopenia in patients receiving heparin therapy.
  - Causes platelet activation, significantly increasing risk of thrombosis.
  - Thrombocytopenia and thrombosis occur 5 – 10 days after exposure to heparin (particularly unfractionated heparin).
  - If HIT is suspected, immediately discontinue heparin and administer anticoagulants.

- **IDIOPATHIC THROMBOCYTOPENIC PURPURA (ITP, IMMUNE THROMBOCYTOPENIA)** is an autoimmune disorder that causes the destruction of platelets.
  - S/s include mild bleeding (e.g., petechiae, purpura); severe GI bleeding and hematuria are more rare.
  - Treatment includes corticosteroids and IVIG.

HELPFUL HINT

Heparin is neutralized with protamine sulfate. Warfarin is neutralized with Vitamin K.

QUICK REVIEW QUESTION

4. A patient with sepsis after a complicated PE has been in the ICU for 2 weeks. The nurse calls the physician because the patient has frank blood in the stool and is oozing from around the PICC lines. Why should the nurse consider thrombocytopenia as the cause?

Sickle Cell Disease
PATHOPHYSIOLOGY

SICKLE CELL DISEASE is an inherited form of hemolytic anemia that causes deformities in the shape of the RBCs. When oxygen levels in the venous circulation are low, the RBCs dehydrate and form a sickle shape. This process can be exacerbated by exposure to cold temperatures or high altitudes. Sickle cell disease is a chronic disease that can lead to complications that require emergency care.

- SICKLE CELL CRISIS (also called vaso-occlusive pain): sickle-shaped cells clump together and restrict blood flow, causing localized ischemia, inflammation, and severe pain.

- ACUTE CHEST SYNDROME (ACS): vaso-occlusion in the lungs (often after an infection) that results in chest pain and respiratory distress.

- APLASTIC CRISIS: anemia that occurs after an infection, usually by human parvovirus; rapid decline of hemoglobin caused by the inability of the bone marrow to produce new cells.

- SPLENIC SEQUESTRATION: pooling of RBCs in the spleen; can lead to anemia and hypovolemia.

- INFECTION: the leading cause of death for children with sickle cell disease; common infections include bacteremia, pneumonia, and osteomyelitis.

- ACUTE INFARCTIONS: blood clots caused by clumped sickle-shaped cells; can lead to hypoxia and infarction (MI, stroke, PE, DVT, etc.).

- PRIAPISM: a common complication for men with sickle cell disease.

DID YOU KNOW?
In the U.S., most diagnoses of sickle cell trait are made following newborn screenings.

TREATMENT AND MANAGEMENT

- treatment based on patient's signs and symptoms

- transfusion of packed RBCs for ACS, splenic sequestration, and symptomatic anemia

- ACS: IV fluids, analgesics, oxygen, low-molecular-weight heparin, hydroxyurea

- sickle cell crisis: analgesics (usually IV opioids)

- standard treatment protocols for other complications (e.g., DVT, priapism, infection)

QUICK REVIEW QUESTION

5. A 26-year-old male with a history of sickle cell disease arrives at the ED with fever, jaundice, and priapism. What symptom is most urgent to address?

DISSEMINATED INTRAVASCULAR COAGULATION (DIC)

PATHOPHYSIOLOGY

DISSEMINATED INTRAVASCULAR COAGULOPATHY (DIC) is a coagulation disorder with simultaneous intervals of clotting and bleeding. Micro clots cascade throughout the vascular system, causing hypoxia and ischemia to multiple organs. In response to these clots, fibrinogens release profuse amounts of anti-clotting factors, triggering both internal and external hemorrhages. DIC may present as acute or chronic:

- **ACUTE (DECOMPENSATED) DIC**: characterized by severe bleeding.
- **CHRONIC (COMPENSATED) DIC**: more likely to lead to thrombosis than to bleeding; can be asymptomatic.

DIAGNOSIS

- s/s of bleeding (e.g., spontaneous hemorrhage, petechiae)
- s/s of thromboembolic event (e.g., PE, DVT)
- acute DIC
  - decreased platelets (moderate to severe) and fibrinogen
  - prolonged PT and PTT
  - severely elevated D-dimer and FSP
- chronic DIC
  - decreased platelets (mild)
  - normal or slightly prolonged PT and PTT
  - normal or slightly decreased fibrinogen
  - elevated D-dimer and FSP

TREATMENT AND MANAGEMENT

- identify and treat underlying cause
- IV fluid resuscitation
- vasopressors
- transfusion of blood products (FFP, PRBCs, platelets, or cryoprecipitate)
- heparin for chronic DIC

QUICK REVIEW QUESTION

6. What diagnostic findings would confirm a diagnosis of acute DIC in a patient recovering from postpartum hemorrhage?

ELECTROLYTE/FLUID IMBALANCE

ELECTROLYTES are positively or negatively charged ions located in both the intracellular fluid (ICF) and the extracellular fluid (ECF). These ions are necessary for the maintenance of homeostasis, cellular excitability, and the transmission of neural impulses.

Table 9.1. Electrolyte Imbalances

IMBALANCE	CLINICAL MANIFESTATION	TREATMENT AND MANAGEMENT	ETIOLOGY
SODIUM (NORMAL: 135 – 145 mEq/L)			
Hyponatremia	• tachycardia • hypotension • weakness • dizziness • headache • abdominal cramping • cerebral edema • increased ICP	• sodium replacement, ≤ 12 mEq/L in a 24-hour period • PO sodium replacement as tolerated • isotonic IV solutions (lactated Ringers or 0.9% normal saline) • restrict fluid intake, and monitor fluid I/O	• dilutional • depletion of Na$^+$ • CHF • diarrhea • diaphoresis • use of thiazides
Hypernatremia	• hypotension • tachycardia • polydipsia • lethargy or irritability • edema • warm, flushed skin • hyperreflexia • seizures	• restrict dietary sodium • increase PO fluid or free-water intake • diuretics • D5W or other hypotonic IV solutions	• sodium overload • volume depletion • impaired thirst • renal or GI loss • inability to replace fluid losses
POTASSIUM (NORMAL: 3.5 – 5 mEq/L)			

Hypokalemia	• dysrhythmias:
	  • flat or inverted T waves
	  • prominent U waves
	  • ST depression
	  • prolonged PR interval
	  • hypotension
	• altered mental status
	• leg cramps or muscle cramps
	• hypoactive reflexes
	• flaccid muscles
		• potassium replacement PO or IV
		• IV administration ≤ 20 mEq/hr
		• stop infusion if urine output < 30 mL/hr
		• cardiac monitoring necessary
		• presents with hypercalcemia
			• acid-base shifts
			• alkalosis
			• true depletion or deficits
			• IV dextrose use
			• diarrhea
			• alcoholism
			• Cushing's syndrome
			• medications: steroids, diuretics, amphotericin, insulin

Hyperkalemia	• dysrhythmias or cardiac arrest:
	  • tall, peaked T waves
	  • prolonged PR interval
	  • wide QRS complex
	  • absent P waves
	  • ST depression
	• abdominal cramping and diarrhea
	• anxiety
		• medication or IV solution, depending on severity of symptoms
		• calcium gluconate
		• IV insulin and D50
		• loop diuretics
		• sodium polystyrene sulfonate (Kayexalate)
		• sodium bicarbonate
		• beta 2 agonists (albuterol)
		• hypertonic IV solution (3% normal saline)
		• ECG and continued cardiac monitoring
		• restrict PO intake of potassium-containing foods
		• may require dialysis
			• increased intake of salt substitutes or potassium-sparing medications
			• hemolysis, burns, crushing injury, or rhabdomyolysis
			• decreased urine output

Table 9.1. Electrolyte Imbalances (continued)

IMBALANCE	CLINICAL MANIFESTATION	TREATMENT AND MANAGEMENT	ETIOLOGY
MAGNESIUM (NORMAL: 1.3 – 2.1 mEq/L)			
Hypo-magnesemia	<ul><li>dysrhythmias:<ul><li>torsades de pointes</li><li>flat or inverted T waves</li><li>ST depression</li><li>prolonged PR interval</li><li>widened QRS complex</li></ul></li><li>hypertension</li><li>Chvostek sign</li><li>Trousseau sign</li><li>seizures</li><li>hyperreflexia</li></ul>	<ul><li>magnesium sulfate IV, 1 – 2 g over 60 minutes</li><li>monitor for seizures, dysrhythmias, and magnesium toxicity</li></ul>	<ul><li>excessive loss from GI tract or kidneys</li><li>diuretic use</li><li>alcoholism</li></ul>
Hyper-magnesemia	<ul><li>dysrhythmias or cardiac arrest:<ul><li>prolonged PR interval</li><li>wide QRS complex</li><li>peaked T waves</li><li>bradycardia (more common) or tachycardia</li></ul></li><li>bradypnea</li><li>respiratory paralysis</li><li>altered mental status, lethargy, or coma</li></ul>	<ul><li>calcium gluconate</li><li>loop diuretics</li><li>isotonic IV solutions (lactated Ringers or 0.9% normal saline)</li><li>may require dialysis</li></ul>	<ul><li>increased intake</li><li>renal dysfunction</li><li>hepatitis</li><li>Addison's disease</li></ul>
CALCIUM (NORMAL: 4.5 – 5.5 mEq/L)			
Hypocalcemia	<ul><li>dysrhythmias or cardiac arrest:<ul><li>prolonged QT interval</li><li>flattened ST segment</li></ul></li><li>hypotension</li><li>third-space fluid shift</li><li>decreased clotting time</li><li>laryngeal spasm or bronchospasm</li><li>seizures</li><li>Chvostek sign</li><li>Trousseau sign</li><li>hyperactive deep-tendon reflexes</li></ul>	<ul><li>PO or IV calcium replacement</li><li>calcium gluconate, 10 – 20 mL, over 5 – 10 minutes</li><li>dilute IV solution with D5W only, never with normal saline</li><li>vitamin D supplements</li><li>seizure precautions</li></ul>	<ul><li>low serum proteins</li><li>decreased intake</li><li>renal failure</li><li>hypoparathyroidism</li><li>vitamin D deficiency</li><li>pancreatitis</li><li>medications: calcitonin, steroids, loop diuretics</li></ul>

IMBALANCE	CLINICAL MANIFESTATION	TREATMENT AND MANAGEMENT	ETIOLOGY
Calcium (normal: 4.5 – 5.5 mEq/L) (continued)			
Hypercalcemia	• anxiety • cognitive dysfunction • constipation • nausea/vomiting • shortened QT interval • muscle weakness	• loop diuretics • isotonic IV solutions (0.9% normal saline) • glucocorticoids and calcitonin	• malignancies • hyperthyroidism and hyperparathyroidism • Paget's disease • medications: lithium, androgens, tamoxifen, excessive vitamin D, excessive thyroid replacement therapy
Phosphate (normal: 1.8 – 2.3 mEq/L)			
Hypo-phosphatemia	• respiratory distress or failure • tissue hypoxia • chest pain • seizures • decreased LOC • increased susceptibility to infection • nystagmus	• PO or IV phosphate replacement • seizure precautions	• increased renal excretion
Hyper-phosphatemia	• tachycardia • Chvostek sign • Trousseau sign • hyperreflexia • soft-tissue calcifications	• saline and loop diuretics • phosphate binders (e.g., aluminum hydroxide) • limit dietary intake of phosphates • dialysis may be appropriate	• decreased renal excretion

Quick Review Question

7. A patient receiving enteral feedings has had severe diarrhea. The patient becomes irritable and is twitching. The nurse's assessment reveals the following vital signs: BP 92/53 mm Hg, HR 108 bpm, RR 20 breaths/min, and oral temperature 38.3°C (100.9°F). What condition should the nurse suspect?

ENDOCRINE CONDITIONS

Acute Adrenal Crisis (Addisonian Crisis)

PATHOPHYSIOLOGY

ACUTE ADRENAL INSUFFICIENCY (ADDISONIAN CRISIS) occurs when the adrenal cortex cannot produce enough corticosteroids to meet the body's needs. It is usually an acute escalation of preexisting adrenal insufficiency but can also be caused by trauma to the adrenal glands. Acute adrenal crisis is rapid onset, causes shock, and requires immediate treatment.

DIAGNOSIS

- dehydration
- hypotension
- hyperpigmentation
- nausea, vomiting, or abdominal pain
- weakness, fatigue, or dizziness
- tachycardia
- respiratory distress
- history of weight loss, anorexia, and/or craving for salt
- electrolyte imbalances: hyperkalemia, hyponatremia, hypercalcemia
- hypoglycemia
- increased serum BUN, serum creatinine
- decreased serum cortisol

TREATMENT AND MANAGEMENT

- treatment based on clinical appearance and not delayed pending diagnostic test results
- IV fluids
- IV corticosteroids
- oxygen; mechanical ventilation if needed

QUICK REVIEW QUESTION

8. A 19-year-old patient who has recently stopped a course of prednisone for asthma exacerbation arrives at the ED with a blood pressure of 78/40 mm Hg, a HR of 135 bpm, fatigue, and extreme thirst. What classification of medication does the nurse anticipate giving this patient?

Hyperglycemia

PATHOPHYSIOLOGY

HYPERGLYCEMIA occurs when serum glucose concentrations are elevated in response to a decrease in available insulin or to insulin resistance. The condition is most often associated with diabetes mellitus but can also be caused by medications (such as corticosteroids and amphetamines), infection, sepsis, and endocrine disorders.

DIABETIC KETOACIDOSIS (DKA) is a hyperglycemic state characterized by an insulin deficiency that stimulates the breakdown of adipose tissues. This process results in the production of ketones and leads to metabolic acidosis. DKA develops quickly (< 24 hours) and is most common in people with type 1 diabetes.

HYPEROSMOLAR HYPERGLYCEMIC STATE (HHS) is a severe hyperglycemic state characterized by profound hyperosmolarity and the absence of acidosis. HHS develops gradually over days to weeks. Volume depletion occurs as the result of osmotic diuresis caused by prolonged hyperglycemia. HHS is more common in persons with type 2 diabetes and has a much higher mortality rate than does DKA.

HHS was previously referred to as hyperosmolar hyperglycemic nonketotic coma (HHNC). The name of the condition changed to reflect that coma is not always present in HHS, although mental status changes and seizures are common.

DIAGNOSIS

Table 9.2. Diagnosis of Diabetic Ketoacidosis (DKA) and Hyperosmolar Hyperglycemic State (HHS)		
	DKA	**HHS**
SIGNS AND SYMPTOMS	• rapid onset • polyuria (early); oliguria (late) • s/s of hypovolemia • Kussmaul respirations • fruity breath odor • polyphagia and polydipsia • nausea, vomiting, and abdominal pain • malaise and weakness • decreased LOC	• slow onset • polyuria • s/s of hypovolemia • rapid, extremely shallow breaths • polydipsia • mild nausea or vomiting • weight loss • diplopia • malaise, weakness, stupor, or coma
DIAGNOSTIC FINDINGS	• elevated blood glucose (> 250 mg/dL) • metabolic acidosis • increased serum ketones • low serum Na^+ and Ca^{++} • increased serum K^+ • elevated BUN and creatinine	• elevated blood glucose (> 600 mg/dL) • high serum osmolality (> 350 mOsm/kg) • serum K^+ normal or high • elevated BUN and creatinine

- IV fluid protocols
  - first hour: 1 – 3 L of isotonic fluids (lactated Ringers or 0.9% normal saline)
  - second hour: 1 L of hypotonic fluids (0.45% normal saline)
  - when blood glucose reaches 250 mg/dL: 1 L of hypertonic fluids with dextrose (D5 in ½ normal saline).
- IV K+ replacement if K+ < 5.3 mEq/L
- continuous IV insulin (0.1 units/kg/hr) when K+ > 3.3 mEq/L
- HHNK may require high-dose insulin due to type 2 DM insulin resistance
- monitoring: cardiac, blood glucose

HELPFUL HINT

For fluid resuscitation in DKA, think "Oh, Oh, Ease off": IsOtonic, hypOtonic, hypErtonic.

QUICK REVIEW QUESTION

9. What diagnostic findings differentiate HHS from DKA?

Hypoglycemia

PATHOPHYSIOLOGY

DID YOU KNOW?
Decreased glucose levels trigger the release of adrenaline (epinephrine) to restore normal glucose levels, leading to increased sympathetic nervous system activity.

HYPOGLYCEMIA occurs when blood sugar (glucose) concentrations fall below normal. Patients will typically show symptoms when serum glucose is < 70 mg/dL, but the onset of symptoms will depend on the patient's tolerance. Common causes of hypoglycemia include use of insulin, adrenal insufficiency, infection, pancreatitis, and excessive vomiting.

DIAGNOSIS

- serum glucose < 70 mg/dL
- tachycardia
- diaphoresis
- irritability, restlessness
- cool skin
- lethargy and weakness
- slurred speech or blurred vision
- anxiety or confusion
- seizure (at blood glucose 20 – 40 mg/dL)
- coma (at blood glucose < 20 mg/dL)

HELPFUL HINT
Beta blockers may hide cardiovascular symptoms in patients with hypoglycemia.

TREATMENT AND MANAGEMENT

- blood glucose 60 – 70 mg/dL: 4 oz of juice if oral intake is not contraindicated
- blood glucose 40 – 60 mg/dL: D50 via IV push (12.5 g = 0.5 ampule)
- blood glucose < 40 mg/dL: D50 via IV push (25 g = 1.0 ampule)
- refractory hypoglycemia: continuous infusion of D10 or D20

QUICK REVIEW QUESTION

10. The nurse is called to a patient care unit to assist with a rapid response. A patient has been found unresponsive, with a blood sugar of 38 mg/dL. What nursing intervention is priority?

Thyrotoxic Crisis

PATHOPHYSIOLOGY

THYROTOXIC CRISIS (THYROID STORM) is a rapid increase in circulating thyroid hormones. The surge in hormones speeds up metabolism in all body systems and increases oxygen demand. Thyrotoxic crisis is the result of untreated or undertreated hyperthyroidism and is a lift-threatening emergency that requires immediate medical intervention.

DIAGNOSIS

- hyperpyrexia
- tachycardia
- respiratory distress
- agitation, delirium, or manic state
- nausea, vomiting, diarrhea, or abdominal pain
- ophthalmopathy
- stupor or coma
- decreased TSH
- elevated free T4, total T4 and T3

TREATMENT AND MANAGEMENT

- treatment based on clinical appearance and not delayed pending thyroid study results
- medications
  - □ beta blocker (propranolol)
  - □ thionamide (prevents synthesis of thyroid hormones)
  - □ iodine
  - □ glucocorticoid
- cooling measures, including antipyretics
- oxygen; mechanical ventilation if needed
- IV fluids

QUICK REVIEW QUESTION

11. A patient arrives at the ED in a thyrotoxic crisis. What therapeutic interventions can the nurse initiate to reduce core body temperature while waiting for antipyretics to take effect?

FEVER ✱

PATHOPHYSIOLOGY

FEVER is an elevation in core body temperature (one-time temperature of 101°F (38.3°C) or any temperature > 100.4°F (38°C) for > 1 hour). Core body temperature is mediated by the thermostatic set point in the thermoregulatory center of the hypothalamus. Fever occurs when the thermostatic set point resets to a higher value in response to circulating pyrogens and cytokines.

The hypothalamus will not raise the body temperature above 105.8°F (41°C). Fevers higher than this indicate damage to the thermoregulatory center and may result from seizure activity, hyperthermic states, and cerebral injuries. All fevers increase the metabolic rate and oxygen consumption.

DIAGNOSIS

- one-time temperature of 101°F (38.3°C)
- temperature of > 100.4°F (38°C) for > 1 hour
- workup for fever of unknown origin:
  - ☐ CBC with differential
  - ☐ blood cultures and serum lactate
  - ☐ ESR
  - ☐ CMP
  - ☐ urinalysis
  - ☐ screen for tuberculosis, HIV
  - ☐ CXR
  - ☐ possible CT scan of abdomen or head
  - ☐ possible lumbar puncture

TREATMENT AND MANAGEMENT

- antipyretics (aspirin contraindicated for pediatric patients)
- cooling techniques
  - ☐ hypothermia blanket
  - ☐ ice packs to armpits, groin, forehead, and back of neck
  - ☐ adjust environmental temperature
  - ☐ minimize patient's clothing and bedding
- IV fluids and oxygen as needed
- identify and treat underlying cause

QUICK REVIEW QUESTION

12. A 4-week-old infant arrives at the ED with lethargy and fever (temperature of 104.5°F [40.3°C]). What diagnostics should the nurse anticipate?

IMMUNOCOMPROMISE

PATHOPHYSIOLOGY

Immune deficiencies can be primary disorders (i.e., inherited) or secondary to disease, medications, or malnutrition. Immune deficiencies commonly seen in emergency care are discussed below.

- **LEUKOPENIA** is the general term for a WBC < 4000/μL. It can occur as the result of impaired production or rapid use of WBCs.

- **ACQUIRED IMMUNODEFICIENCY SYNDROME (AIDS)** is the end-stage progression of HIV. Patients with AIDS have a depletion of T lymphocytes and are susceptible to opportunistic and sometimes emergent infections.

- **LEUKEMIA,** cancer of the WBCs, occurs in the bone marrow and disrupts the production and function of WBCs. In the absence of functioning

WBCs, the patient becomes immunocompromised. The types of leukemia are differentiated by which WBCs are affected (lymphocytes or myeloid cells).

- **CHEMOTHERAPY** is conducted with a class of cytotoxic medications that destroy cancer cells by disrupting cell mitosis and DNA replication. A side effect of chemotherapy is severe **NEUTROPENIA** (a decrease in circulating neutrophils).

- Poorly managed **DIABETES MELLITUS**, and associated hyperglycemia, increases the risk of infection. In the critical care setting, patients with diabetes are more prone to postoperative infections and skin infections.

TREATMENT AND MANAGEMENT

- treat patient's complaints and symptoms, usually fever and infection
- specialized care to prevent opportunistic infections
  - ☐ appropriate precautions for patient, providers, and visitors
  - ☐ maintain patient skin integrity
  - ☐ ensure adequate nutrition and hydration
  - ☐ prophylactic antibiotics

QUICK REVIEW QUESTION

13. A patient receiving chemotherapy presents with onset of cough and fever. A CBC reveals a WBC count of 20,000/µL and a left shift. Blood cultures are drawn, with results pending, and the patient's lactic acid level is 2.9 mmol/L. Chest X-ray shows bilateral pulmonary infiltrates. What diagnosis does the nurse anticipate?

RENAL FAILURE

PATHOPHYSIOLOGY

ACUTE KIDNEY INJURY (AKI), also called acute renal failure, is an acute decrease in kidney function characterized by increased serum creatinine (**AZOTEMIA**) with or without decreased urine output. Changes in kidney function may result in multiple systemic conditions that require intervention. These conditions include fluid, electrolyte, and acid-base imbalance and hematological abnormalities (e.g., anemia, low platelet count).

AKI has a diverse etiology and is characterized as prerenal, intrarenal, or postrenal, based on the cause of injury.

- **PRERENAL DISEASE** is renal hypoperfusion caused by hemodynamic compromise (e.g., hypovolemia, systemic vasodilation) or renal ischemia. It is usually reversed by treating the underlying condition.
  - ☐ Diagnosis: increased creatinine and BUN; elevated BUN-to-creatinine ratio (> 20:1); low urine Na^+; increased urine osmolality and specific gravity; normal finding on urine microscopy (no casts); serum creatinine returns to normal value after fluid repletion

□ Management: treat underlying cause to maintain MAP > 65 mm Hg; fluids to rehydrate; vasopressors as needed to manage vasodilation

■ **INTRARENAL** (intrinsic) **DISEASE** is caused by damage to the kidneys. The most common intrarenal condition is **ACUTE TUBULAR NECROSIS (ATN)**, the destruction of the renal tubular epithelium, which may be ischemic or nephrotoxic.

□ Diagnosis: increased creatinine and BUN; BUN-to-creatinine ratio < 20:1; increase or decrease in urine osmolality and specific gravity (depending on phase of disease); low urine Na⁺; casts seen through urine microscopy; serum creatinine does not respond to fluid repletion

□ Management: treat underlying cause; discontinue or minimize use of nephrotoxic medications; IV fluids for hypovolemia; loop diuretics for hypervolemia; correct electrolyte imbalances; monitor for related complications; sodium bicarbonate for metabolic acidosis; monitor for indications for urgent dialysis (severe or symptomatic hyperkalemia, severe metabolic acidosis, volume overload, pulmonary edema, uremia)

■ **POSTRENAL CONDITIONS** are characterized by the blocked drainage of urine, usually because of prostatic hypertrophy or renal calculi.

□ Diagnosis: oliguria; increased serum creatinine and BUN; normal BUN-to-creatinine ratio; possible pain or hematuria

□ Management: treat underlying cause of obstruction

QUICK REVIEW QUESTION

14. A patient with sepsis has received 3 L of normal saline over the past 24 hours and currently has maintenance fluids at 125 mL/hr. The nurse notes that urine output is at 250 mL for the past 4 hours. The last serum creatinine is 1.8 mg/dL, and BUN is 38 mg/dL. What interventions should the nurse anticipate?

★ SEPSIS AND SEPTIC SHOCK

PATHOPHYSIOLOGY

SEPSIS, a massive inflammatory response to systemic infection, can lead to multi-organ failure and death. The most common sites of initial infection are blood (bacteremia), the lungs (pneumonia), the urinary tract or kidneys, and the abdominal area (e.g., peritonitis or ruptured appendix). Sepsis progresses through 4 stages:

1. systemic inflammatory response syndrome (SIRS)

2. sepsis

3. severe sepsis

4. septic shock

MULTIPLE ORGAN DYSFUNCTION SYNDROME (MODS) refers to the dysfunction of one or more organs and requires supportive therapy in an acute illness. MODS is sometimes placed on the most severe end of the sepsis spectrum.

DIAGNOSIS

Table 9.3. Diagnosis of Sepsis Conditions			
SIRS	**SEPSIS**	**SEVERE SEPSIS**	**SEPTIC SHOCK**
• temperature > 101°F (38.3°C) or < 96.9°F (36°C) • HR > 90 bpm • RR > 20 per minute • $PaCO_2$ < 32 mm Hg • WBC > 12,000/mm³ or < 4,000/mm³ or > 10% bands	• 2 or more signs or symptoms of SIRS, plus suspected or confirmed infection • serum lactate > 2 mmol/L	• sepsis, plus new or acute onset of organ dysfunction • urine output <30 cc/h • altered mental status • respiratory distress • tachycardia • abdominal pain • systolic BP < 90 mm Hg • MAP < 60 mm Hg • serum lactate >4 mmol/L • thrombocytopenia • elevated liver enzymes	severe sepsis, plus persistent hypotension and hypoperfusion that does not respond to fluid volume replacement

TREATMENT AND MANAGEMENT

- oxygen; mechanical ventilation as needed
- IV fluids: 30 mL/kg in rapidly infused boluses
- broad-spectrum antibiotics
- vasopressors

QUICK REVIEW QUESTION

15. A patient with septic shock has a blood pressure of 84/38 mg Hg after receiving a 1 L normal saline bolus. What medication should the nurse anticipate administering?

ANSWER KEY

1. Loratadine is an H1 blocker. H2 blockers, glucocorticoids, bronchodilators, and topical antihistamines will also help reduce the allergic response to poison ivy.

2. The nurse should expect to administer epinephrine 1:1,000 IM 0.01 mg/kg.

3. Factor VIII transfusion should be initiated immediately if not previously started by the parent or school nurse.

4. The patient would have been administered heparin to treat the PE, so heparin-induced thrombocytopenia should be considered as a cause of the bleeding.

5. Priapism can lead to permanent impotence, sexual dysfunction, and tissue necrosis. This symptom requires immediate treatment to restore blood flow.

6. Obstetrical complications are a common cause of DIC. Diagnostic findings that would confirm this diagnosis include thrombocytopenia, prolonged clotting times (PT and PTT), decreased fibrinogen, and increased levels of fibrinolysis products (D-dimer and FSP).

7. The patient's history and symptoms suggest hypernatremia, likely due to the dehydration associated with diarrhea and possibly insufficient free water administered with the enteral feedings.

8. The patient will likely receive IV corticosteroids to treat Addisonian crisis related to the abrupt discontinuation of the prednisone.

9. The preferred diagnostic indicator is serum osmolality: patients with HHS will have a higher serum osmolality (> 350 mOsm/kg) than with DKA. HHS also presents with higher blood glucose (> 600 mg/dL) than DKA. Because no ketoacidosis is present with HHS, there will be no significant serum ketones or findings associated with acidosis.

10. The patient needs glucose immediately: establish IV access, and push 1 ampule of D50.

11. The nurse can use a hypothermia blanket, can apply ice packs to the armpits and groin and behind the neck, and can reduce the room temperature.

12. Workup for fever of unknown origin in an infant includes CBC, blood cultures, chest X-ray, urinalysis, and possible lumbar puncture.

13. The nurse should suspect septic pneumonia. Chemotherapy immunocompromises patients, making them more susceptible to infection.

14. The patient is likely experiencing sepsis-induced prerenal disease. The nurse should ensure optimal perfusion through continued fluid replacement and titrating vasopressors to keep MAP > 65 mm Hg. The physician should be notified if the patient does not respond with improving urine output.

15. Vasopressors such as dobutamine hydrochloride, norepinephrine (Levophed), and phenylephrine hydrochloride (Neo-Synephrine) are used for supportive therapy of organ perfusion related to hypotension.

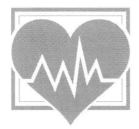

MAXILLOFACIAL EMERGENCIES

PERITONSILLAR ABSCESS

PATHOPHYSIOLOGY

PERITONSILLAR ABSCESS is an acute medical emergency that compromises the airway. Purulent exudate accumulates between the tonsillar capsule and the pharyngeal constrictor muscle causing cellulitis and edema. This is a life-threatening condition that can quickly advance to mediastinitis, intracranial abscess, necrotizing fasciitis, streptococcal toxic shock syndrome, and empyema if the infection is not aggressively managed.

DIAGNOSIS

- visible abscess on soft palate
- severe sore throat
- enlarged lymph nodes

- fever
- trismus
- drooling
- dysphagia
- halitosis
- labs show infection

TREATMENT AND MANAGEMENT

- maintain airway
- analgesics, antibiotics, and/or corticosteroids
- incision and drainage or needle aspiration

QUICK REVIEW QUESTION

1. An 18-year-old patient arrives at the ED with a complaint of sore throat, drooling, and severe halitosis that the nurse can detect from several feet away. In the triage setting, what can the nurse immediately assess for to determine the level of acuity for this patient?

DENTAL CONDITIONS

PATHOPHYSIOLOGY

Emergency dental conditions commonly seen in the ED are dental traumas, abscessed teeth, and acute dental pain.

DIAGNOSIS

- trauma: fractured or cracked tooth, dental avulsion, or lacerations
- abscess/infection: orofacial edema, halitosis, pus or exudate in mouth, general s/s of infection
- dental pain: limited diagnosis in ED, based on patient complaint

TREATMENT AND MANAGEMENT

- trauma
  - analgesics and ice to the face for pain management
  - avulsed tooth placed in Hank's balanced salt solution (HBSS) or milk
  - reinsertion of tooth if viable
  - fracture stabilization and suture repair as needed
- abscess/infection
  - incision and drainage
  - antibiotics, analgesics
- dental pain: analgesics and dental/oral surgery consult

2. A patient arrives at the ED with a complaint of severe mouth pain for the past three days. Assessment findings include edematous gingivitis, an enlarged spongy nodule with purulent yellow exudate along the bottom left molars, facial edema, and tender lymph nodes. What is the diagnosis and why is medical care important?

EPISTAXIS

PATHOPHYSIOLOGY

EPISTAXIS is hemorrhage or bleeding in the nasal passages caused by rupture of vasodilated vessels in the mucous membranes. Rupture can occur in one or more vessels and more commonly presents unilaterally. Emergency treatment should be considered if bleeding cannot be self-controlled or compromises the airway. Epistaxis can occur frequently in some individuals and rarely requires emergency management.

DIAGNOSIS

- visible frank bleeding from nares
- facial X-ray for injury

TREATMENT AND MANAGEMENT

- manage airway
- position patient sitting upright and leaning forward to prevent aspiration
- continuous pressure to midline septum by pinching with fingers for up to 15 minutes
- ice for pain management and vasoconstriction
- nasal decongestant spray for vasoconstriction
- nasal packing if bleeding continues

HELPFUL HINT

Do not have patients with epistaxis tilt their head backward because it can direct blood to the airway.

QUICK REVIEW QUESTION

3. A patient arrives in the ED with acute epistaxis after being hit with a football in the face during a high school game. The patient suddenly goes into respiratory distress. What actions should the nurse take immediately?

FACIAL NERVE DISORDERS

Bell's Palsy

PATHOPHYSIOLOGY

BELL'S PALSY is a unilateral facial paralysis or weakness caused by inflammation of the facial nerve (seventh cranial nerve). Onset is sudden and facial droop is similar in appearance to droop present with a cerebrovascular accident. In most cases the weakness will resolve over weeks to months; occasionally, it may recur.

Bell's palsy typically occurs in younger adults and children. Cause is unknown but may be related to viral infections, autoimmune disease, or vascular ischemia.

DIAGNOSIS

- mild to total unilateral paralysis of facial muscles
- characteristic facial droop
- painful sensations on affected side
- difficulty speaking
- dysphagia

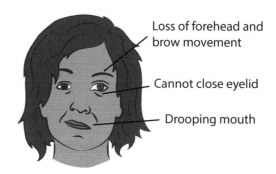

Loss of forehead and brow movement

Cannot close eyelid

Drooping mouth

Figure 10.1. Bell's Palsy

TREATMENT AND MANAGEMENT

- initial diagnostics to rule out CVA
- corticosteroids
- antivirals if indicated
- patch on affected eye if diminished blink reflex to limit risk for corneal abrasion
- oral glycerin swabs for dry mouth
- Yankauer suction for excess saliva
- referral to neurology if warranted

QUICK REVIEW QUESTION

4. A 14-year-old patient arrives at the ED with sudden onset of right-sided facial droop. The patient reveals a recent influenza infection, and Bell's palsy is the suspected diagnosis. What treatment should the nurse anticipate giving this patient?

Trigeminal Neuralgia

PATHOPHYSIOLOGY

TRIGEMINAL NEURALGIA—or tic douloureux—is a condition of the trigeminal nerve (fifth cranial nerve) that causes unilateral stabbing, shooting pain and burning sensations along the nerve branches. Painful spasms both start and end abruptly. Paroxysms can affect any or all of the three nerve branches: ophthalmic, maxillary, and mandibular. The cause is unknown, but pressure and compression of the vascular vessels near the trigeminal nerve root is suspected.

Trigeminal neuralgia is chronic, and the slightest touch or stimulation may precipitate a painful episode. The initial attacks may be short; however, it can progress to longer and more frequent attacks.

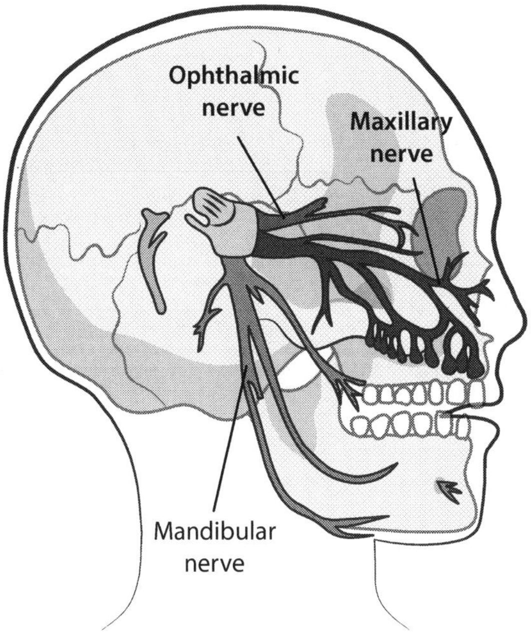

DIAGNOSIS

- characteristic unilateral pain along branches of the fifth cranial nerve
- abrupt onset and ending of pain lasting several minutes to several days
- facial muscle contractions causing eye to close and mouth to twitch on affected side

TREATMENT AND MANAGEMENT

- initial diagnostics to rule out CVA
- anti-seizure medications: carbamazepine (Tegretol), gabapentin (Neurontin), phenytoin (Dilantin)
- neurology consult

Figure 10.2. The Trigeminal Nerve

QUICK REVIEW QUESTION

5. A 50-year-old female patient arrives at the ED with a complaint of excruciating pain when anything touches her face and when eating, brushing her teeth, and putting on makeup. Her symptoms have evolved over the past few weeks. Her medical history includes possible multiple sclerosis. She could not tolerate being touched for the physical assessment and made it partway through the neurological exam. What diagnosis and treatment should the nurse anticipate?

FOREIGN BODIES IN THE NASAL AND ORAL ORIFICES

PATHOPHYSIOLOGY

NON-PENETRATING FOREIGN BODIES may be present in the orifices of the maxillofacial region as a result of aspiration or direct entry.

- Common foreign bodies in nares: popcorn kernels, beads, batteries, Styrofoam pellets, pebbles, and insects
- Common foreign bodies in ear: earring backings, beads, pebbles, popcorn kernels, and insects

DIAGNOSIS

- visible foreign body or sensation of foreign body
- rhinorrhea; may smell foul if present for a prolonged period

- unilateral edema of alar tissue
- ear pain or pressure
- auditory disturbances
- inflammation/edema in turbinates
- otitis media/externa

TREATMENT AND MANAGEMENT

- manage airway (prevent passage of foreign body through nasopharynx)
- tilt head of bed 45 – 90 degrees
- For objects in the nares
    - 0.5% phenylephrine to reduce nasal inflammation
    - topical lidocaine
    - instruct patient to blow nose while blocking unaffected nostril
    - for small children: have parent blow softly into child's mouth while blocking unaffected nostril
    - forceps or suction catheter for retrieval
- when removing objects from ears: use caution to avoid pushing foreign body deeper into the ear canal
- in the case of insects: insert topical lidocaine alcohol or mineral oil to disable movement, or use a flashlight to draw insect out

QUICK REVIEW QUESTION

6. What noninvasive technique can be used by the nurse to remove a live insect foreign body from the ear canal?

INFINFECTIONS

DID YOU KNOW?
Otitis media is the second most common reason for ED visits in children < 1 year old. (Fever is the most common.)

- **ACUTE OTITIS MEDIA** is inflammation of the middle ear that usually results from inflammation in the mucous membranes. It is one of the most common reasons for ED visits in children.
    - Diagnosis: otalgia; otorrhea; tugging on ear; perforated, opaque, bulging, or erythematous tympanic membrane
    - Management: can heal spontaneously; oral antibiotics if membrane is intact; antibiotic drops in affected ear if membrane is ruptured; analgesics
- **LUDWIG'S ANGINA** is a gangrenous cellulitis in the soft tissue of the neck and the floor of the mouth, generally following dental abscess. Edema in the neck and mouth places the patient at high risk for airway obstruction.
    - Diagnosis: tongue enlargement and protrusion; sublingual pain and tenderness; compromised breathing; difficulty swallowing; drooling; labs and s/s consistent with infection
    - Management: manage airway; IV antibiotics; incision and drainage

- **MASTOIDITIS** is a bacterial infection of the mastoid air cells within the mastoid bone. It typically occurs secondary to acute otitis media.
  - ☐ Diagnosis: otitis media; tympanic membrane rupture; papilledema; erythema and edema over mastoid process
  - ☐ Management: antibiotics; analgesics
- **SINUSITIS** is inflammation and edema of the membranes lining the sinus cavities.
  - ☐ Diagnosis: facial pressure and pain; headache; nasal congestion and blockage; green or yellow nasal discharge
  - ☐ Management: decongestant/antihistamine; analgesics; antibiotics; corticosteroids; humidified air, warm compress, or saline nasal drops

QUICK REVIEW QUESTION

7. A male patient is admitted to the ED one week after oral surgery with pain and swelling to the left side of his face and neck, which has progressed through the day. He states he has had difficulty swallowing and is drooling. He rates the pain 7/10 and vital signs reveal a temperature of 100.0°F (37.8°C) and pulse of 114 bpm. The oral cavity is tender and painful upon palpation. What diagnosis is appropriate for these signs and symptoms, and what test can be ordered to confirm?

ACUTE VESTIBULAR DYSFUNCTION

Labyrinthitis

PATHOPHYSIOLOGY

LABYRINTHITIS occurs in the inner ear when the vestibulocochlear nerve (eighth cranial nerve) becomes inflamed as the result of either bacterial or viral infection. The inflammation affects hearing, balance, and spatial navigation. Onset is characterized as acute, sudden, and painless. The initial episode is most severe, with subsequent episodes showing less intensity. Labyrinthitis symptoms can extend from several weeks to several months.

DIAGNOSIS

- dizziness and vertigo
- nausea and vomiting
- loss of balance
- tinnitus or hearing loss
- imaging/labs to rule out neurological condition, Ménière's disease

TREATMENT AND MANAGEMENT

- antibiotics or antivirals
- corticosteroids
- supportive care for symptoms: antihistamines, antiemetics, benzodiazepines

8. A 40-year-old female is diagnosed with labyrinthitis in the ED after all other potential neurological causes for sudden onset of vertigo, nausea, and tinnitus have been ruled out. While the nurse is preparing the patient for discharge, the patient asks if she can return to work tomorrow. What should the nurse anticipate discussing with the patient about the course of this disease?

Ménière's Disease

PATHOPHYSIOLOGY

MÉNIÈRE'S DISEASE is the result of chronic excess fluid in the inner ear. Fluid accumulation is the result of malabsorption in the endolymphatic sac or blockage of the endolymphatic duct. The excess fluid causes the endolymphatic space to enlarge, increasing inner ear pressure and possibly rupturing the inner membrane (not to be confused with rupture of the tympanic membrane in the middle ear as seen with otitis media).

While typically only one ear is affected, it does occur bilaterally in about 20% of cases. Onset may be minor with subtle symptoms, with subsequent episodes manifesting with more severe symptoms. Attacks can occur frequently, up to several times per week, or infrequently, several months or years apart. Attacks typically last anywhere from 20 minutes to 24 hours.

DIAGNOSIS

- classic triad of symptoms: fluctuations in hearing/hearing loss, tinnitus, vertigo

- pre-attack (aura): loss of balance, dizziness, pressure in ear, hearing loss or tinnitus, headache

- mid-attack: sudden severe vertigo, anxiety, GI symptoms, blurred vision, nystagmus, palpitations

- post-attack: extreme exhaustion and need for sleep

- late-stage disease: permanent hearing loss and increases in balance/visual disturbances

- imaging/labs to rule out neurological condition, labyrinthitis

TREATMENT AND MANAGEMENT

- intratympanic gentamicin and steroids (injected by ENT)

- diuretics (non-potassium-sparing) and reduced sodium diet

- supportive care for symptoms: antihistamines, antiemetics, benzodiazepines

QUICK REVIEW QUESTION

9. A 43-year-old female patient arrives at the ED with a complaint of vertigo and tinnitus lasting >20 minutes. Patient states that the onset was sudden and occurred while she was shopping. Patient states she has had vertigo in the past but never this severe. She denies cold and flu symptoms. Vital signs:

DID YOU KNOW?

Tumarkin's otolithic crisis (drop attacks) occur in the late stages of Ménière's disease. They occur when a sudden loss of balance causes the patient to fall. The patient remains conscious and usually recovers quickly.

temperature of 98.6°F (37.0°C), pulse of 88 bpm, RR 16 BPM, BP 112/74 mm Hg, O$_2$ sat 99% on room air. What key information leads the nurse to suspect Ménière's disease versus labyrinthitis?

RUPTURED TYMPANIC MEMBRANE

PATHOPHYSIOLOGY

The **TYMPANIC MEMBRANE** (eardrum) is a stiff yet flexible structure that separates the ear canal from the middle ear. Any tear or perforation in this membrane is termed a rupture. In uncomplicated cases a ruptured eardrum heals without treatment in a few weeks; complicated cases may require specialized procedures and/or surgery.

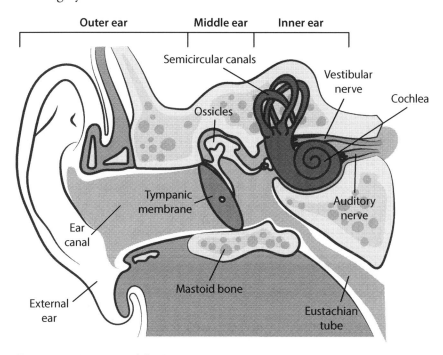

Figure 10.3. Anatomy of the Ear

SIGNS AND SYMPTOMS

- severe pain upon rupture, which quickly subsides
- fluid drainage:
  - clear (effusion)
  - purulent (infection)
  - sanguineous (trauma)
  - serous (suspect cerebrospinal)—emergent
- hearing loss or tinnitus
- vertigo with nausea and vomiting
- whistling sound or crepitus with blowing nose
- rupture visible in otoscope exam

- treatment dependent on root cause of rupture; emergent treatment not always warranted

- antibiotic and/or analgesic ear drops

QUICK REVIEW QUESTION

10. A patient presents to the ED with a complaint of left ear pain following her first time scuba diving. Her medical history is unremarkable and vital signs are stable. The patient states there was an episode of severe pain just as she surfaced. The pain got better, but now she has difficulty hearing. What tool will be used for initial evaluation and what treatment is the patient likely to need?

TEMPOROMANDIBULAR JOINT DISLOCATION

PATHOPHYSIOLOGY

TEMPOROMANDIBULAR JOINT (TMJ) DISLOCATION is a painful condition that can occur related to trauma, excessive opening of the mandible, or force applied to a partially opened mouth. The jaw can dislocate into several positions, including anterior, posterior, superior, and lateral. Anterior displacements are very common and are classified as acute, chronic recurrent, or chronic.

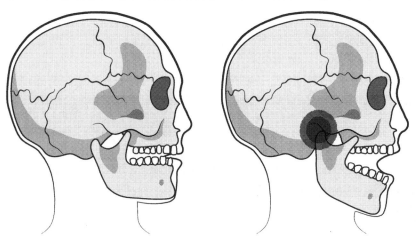

Figure 10.4. Temporomandibular Joint (TMJ) Dislocation

DIAGNOSIS

- palpable displacement of joint

- jaw pain

- malocclusion

- speech difficulties

- drooling

- dysphagia

- trismus

- manage airway

- closed: analgesia and muscle relaxer for manual reduction

- open: surgical treatment or reduction

QUICK REVIEW QUESTION

11. A patient presents to the ED with an anterior TMJ dislocation. The patient states he has jaw pain and trouble swallowing and talking and can feel that his jaw is crooked. What is the nurse's primary assessment and what will be the treatment?

TRAUMA ★

Maxillofacial Fractures

PATHOPHYSIOLOGY

MAXILLOFACIAL FRACTURES occur from both blunt and penetrating traumas. Emergency management focuses on maintaining a patent airway and stabilizing the patient for surgical intervention. Most fractures will involve the integrity of surrounding tissues, requiring complex repair to muscular, vascular, and dermal structures as well as the reduction and fixation of the affected bone.

Types of maxillofacial fractures:

- nasal: most common of all facial fractures and least likely to need specialist consultation

- orbital rim and blowout fractures: fractures of orbital floor or lateral and medial orbital walls; occur from direct blow to the orbit such as from a baseball or fist

- mandibular: fractures of the lower jaw; may be singular or multiple

- maxillary: fractures of the upper jaw

- Le Fort I: horizontal fracture; separates teeth from upper structures—"floating palate"

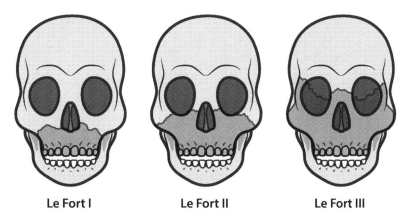

Le Fort I   Le Fort II   Le Fort III

Figure 10.5. Types of Maxillary Fractures

- Le Fort II: pyramidal fracture; teeth are the base of the pyramid, fracture passes diagonally along the lateral wall of the maxillary sinuses, apex of pyramid is the nasofrontal junction—"floating maxilla"

- Le Fort III: craniofacial disjunction transverse fracture line passes through the nasofrontal junction, maxillofrontal suture, orbital wall, zygomatic arch, and zygomatico frontal suture—"floating face"

- Zygomaticomaxillary complex (tripod) fracture: simultaneous fracture of the lateral and inferior orbital rim, the zygomatic arch, and lateral maxillary sinus wall; occurs from direct blow to the lateral cheek

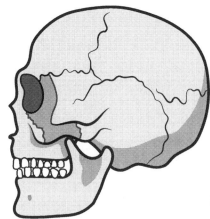

Figure 10.6. Zygomaticomaxillary Complex (Tripod) Fracture

DIAGNOSIS

- visible facial injury or deformity

- pain, tenderness, or paresthesia over affected area

- epistaxis

- ecchymosis

- ocular: diplopia, restricted extraocular movements, decreased vision, enophthalmos, periorbital hematoma or edema, subconjunctival hemorrhage

- dental/oral: visible dental fractures or avulsions, impaired mastication, malocclusion, trismus, rhinorrhea of cerebrospinal fluid

- facial X-ray or CT scan (head and neck)

TREATMENT AND MANAGEMENT

HELPFUL HINT
Cervical spine injuries are seen in around 15 percent of unconscious patients with maxillofacial fractures.

- maintain airway

- cervical spine precautions

- treatment based on type and severity of injury

- goal of all treatments is to preserve function and minimize disfigurement

QUICK REVIEW QUESTION

12. What diagnostic test needs to be performed stat on a patient with a suspected mandibular fracture that presents with dental avulsions?

Soft Tissue Injuries

PATHOPHYSIOLOGY

Penetrative and blunt trauma injuries to the maxillofacial region will cause soft tissue injuries that may obstruct the airway.

DIAGNOSIS

- visible entry wound or foreign object
- bleeding
- contusions, hematoma, or tissue edema
- nasal drainage (rule out cerebrospinal fluid)

TREATMENT AND MANAGEMENT

- priority: maintain airway
- immobilize spine and neck as warranted
- IV fluids as needed for hemorrhage
- apply direct pressure for hemorrhage
- clean or irrigate wounds, then dress
- analgesics
- remove foreign object(s) when it is safe to do so; surgery to remove objects may be required

QUICK REVIEW QUESTION

13. A patient is brought to the ED via ambulance following a hunting accident. A friend states that the patient had lowered the butt of the shotgun to the ground and it accidently fired buckshot into the right side of the patient's neck, chin, and cheek. The patient's neck, face, eye, and mouth exhibit severe swelling and bleeding at entry points, and the patient is unable to speak and has labored breathing. What are the priority steps for the nurse to stabilize this patient?

ANSWER KEY

1. The nurse can use a penlight to assess the tonsillar tissue and soft palate for presence of a peritonsillar abscess. Peritonsillar abscess is an emergent finding and requires rapid evaluation by a medical provider.

2. An abscess is an emergent situation because the infection can spread to the bone and vascular system, causing sepsis and potential death.

3. Suction immediately to maintain patent airway. Sit the patient upright and lean the head forward to prevent aspiration. Ensure pressure is applied to the midline septum to slow the progress of bleeding.

4. The nurse should provide comfort measures to assist with dry eyes, which could include moisture/saline drops and patching to prevent dryness and potential for corneal abrasion. Oral glycerin swabs could be used for dry mouth symptoms, and Yankauer suction can control excess pooling of saliva secretions. Corticosteroids and antiviral medication may be prescribed.

5. Based on signs and symptoms, the patient is suffering from trigeminal neuralgia. The nurse should anticipate pharmacotherapy as a first line of treatment.

6. Some live insects, such as moths, are naturally drawn to light. The nurse can direct a flashlight or exam light into the ear canal to draw the insect outward. This technique may not work if the insect is injured or is trapped in wax or fluid.

7. Signs and symptoms are consistent with early onset of Ludwig's angina. A CT scan to evaluate the soft tissue would be appropriate.

8. Labyrinthitis runs a course of several weeks to several months. The nurse should educate the patient that bedrest is essential and that use of prescribed medications will manage symptoms. It is likely that additional episodes will occur, although they may be less severe than the onset of disease.

9. Ménière's disease presents suddenly with vertigo and tinnitus. While hearing loss can be present, it is common that early attacks lack the typical triad of symptoms. A history of less severe episodes of vertigo is consistent with progressive chronic disease. A patient who is afebrile and denies cold or flu symptoms is likely to have Ménière's disease and not labyrinthitis.

10. An otoscope will be used to assess the tympanic membrane for a tear or hole. For a minor rupture of the eardrum no treatment would be necessary.

11. With facial trauma, the ABCs are priority. A manual reduction is most likely if fractures are ruled out first.

12. The patient should receive a chest X-ray to assess for aspiration of avulsed teeth and bone fragments.

13. This is a traumatic injury with the risk of death. The nurse should start with the ABCs: stabilizing the airway is priority. Prepare for intubation before the airway is lost and administer oxygen or bag patient until airway is secured. Suction oral cavity and start large-bore IVs and fluids for blood loss. Apply direct pressure or pressure bandages to bleeding wounds and administer IV pain medication and sedative. Once the patient is stable, evaluation and removal of buckshot can follow.

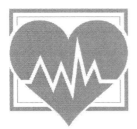

11

OCULAR EMERGENCIES

BCEN CONTENT OUTLINE

✴ **A. ABRASIONS**

   B. Burns

   C. Foreign bodies

✴ **D. GLAUCOMA**

   E. Infections (e.g., conjunctivitis, iritis)

✴ **F. RETINAL ARTERY OCCLUSION**

✴ **G. RETINAL DETACHMENT**

   H. Trauma (e.g., hyphema, laceration, globe rupture)

   I. Ulcerations/keratitis

CORNEAL ABRASION ✴

PATHOPHYSIOLOGY

A **CORNEAL ABRASION** is a scratch or abrasive friction on the outer surface of the epithelium (the cornea's outer layer). Symptoms, severity, and outcome are variable based on the layers of the cornea involved and the size of the area affected. Corneal abrasions typically heal within 24 – 72 hours without complications, but in some cases may progress to infection, keratitis, or ulceration.

SIGNS AND SYMPTOMS

- painful pressure or burning sensation
- sensation of foreign body or grit
- lacrimation or discharge
- erythema or edema
- decrease in visual acuity: may be described as blurred, dull, or foggy

- fluorescein staining
- slit lamp or Woods lamp exam to identify the degree of injury or illness

TREATMENT AND MANAGEMENT

HELPFUL HINT

Do not patch corneal abrasions or lacerations: patching decreases oxygen delivery to the cornea and increases risk of infection.

- irrigate to remove foreign body, if present
- topical anesthetic
- topical antibiotics
- topical NSAIDs
- ophthalmic lubricating solution

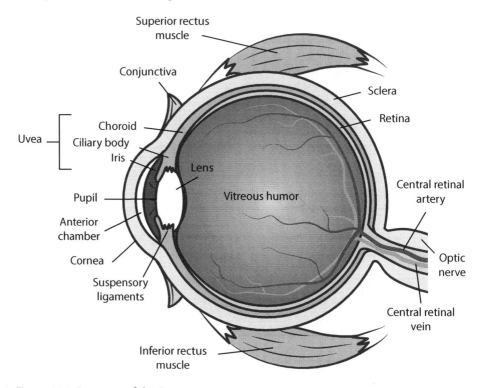

Figure 11.1. Anatomy of the Eye

QUICK REVIEW QUESTION

1. A patient arrives in the ED complaining of a burning sensation in both eyes with increased tearing. The patient states he had "day surgery" for oral tooth extraction about 8 hours ago and noticed the pain shortly after being discharged. The nurse identifies that the pain is bilateral, making the presence of a foreign body unlikely. What diagnostics should the nurse anticipate for this patient?

OCULAR BURNS

PATHOPHYSIOLOGY

OCULAR BURNS are classified as chemical (subdivided as alkali- or acid-based) or radiant energy (thermal or ultraviolet). Chemical burns occur through splash, spray, or direct touch. Alkali burns penetrate deep into the eye, causing liquefactive necrosis, while acidic burns cause a coagulated necrosis closer to the surface of the injury. Radiant energy burns occur from exposure to intense heat, explosions, hot cooking oils, electrical arc, lasers, and direct gaze into ultraviolet light.

The outcome varies based on the agent of exposure, time length of exposure, and ocular structures involved, but usually involves some degree of vision loss. Ocular burns tend to occur bilaterally and often in combination with other injuries such as dermal burns, penetrating objects, and compromised airways.

DIAGNOSIS

- extreme pain or burning sensation
- erythema and edema
- copious lacrimation
- decrease in visual acuity

TREATMENT AND MANAGEMENT

- maintain airway and assess for concurrent injury
- irrigate for minimum of 30 minutes with isotonic solution
  - □ assess pH level after irrigation; if > 7.4, continue with additional irrigation
  - □ topical anesthetics may be added to irrigant solution
  - □ Morgan Lens as needed to assist with irrigation
- topical corticosteroids
- topical antibiotics
- topical cycloplegics
- occlusive dressing as needed
- obtain chemical safety data sheet and consider consultation with regional poison control center

HELPFUL HINT
Irrigation should be deferred if globe rupture is suspected.

QUICK REVIEW QUESTION

2. A 38-year-old male patient arrives at the ED clutching his face after an automobile battery exploded, splashing acidic liquid into his eyes. Irrigation with 1 L normal saline is initiated immediately. How will the nurse assess if the irrigation has been effective or if additional irrigation may be needed?

FOREIGN BODIES IN OCULAR REGION

PATHOPHYSIOLOGY

Ocular foreign bodies are any substance or object that does not belong in the eye. Size, shape, substance, impact velocity, and location will greatly impact severity of symptoms and ultimate outcome.

Foreign bodies are described based upon their location.

- extraocular (lid, sclera, conjunctiva, and cornea)
- intraocular (anterior chamber, iris, lens, vitreous, retina, and intraorbital)

DIAGNOSIS

- visible foreign object
- sensation of foreign body or grit
- painful pressure or burning sensation
- penetrating injury: bleeding
- lacrimation or discharge
- erythema or edema
- blepharospasm
- photosensitivity or decrease in visual acuity
- fluorescein staining
- slit lamp or Woods lamp exam to identify the degree of injury or illness

TREATMENT AND MANAGEMENT

- irrigate with normal saline or eye wash solution
- evert upper lid to confirm absence/presence of foreign body
- Morgan Lens for extraocular foreign bodies, or if sensation of foreign body is present but foreign body is not visible.
- remove foreign body using cotton-tipped applicator, metal spud, or 25-gauge needle (extraocular only)
- topical anesthetic
- topical antibiotics
- topical NSAIDs
- ophthalmic lubricating solution (artificial tears)
- patch if foreign body is retained (pending ophthalmology referral)
- immediate ophthalmology referral for all intraocular foreign bodies

HELPFUL HINT
Ophthalmic corticosteroids are used cautiously and only by ophthalmologists as they can worsen underlying infections in the eye.

QUICK REVIEW QUESTION

3. A patient in a small community hospital is diagnosed with a retained foreign body to the left lens with vitreous leakage present. The patient will require transfer to a larger hospital for emergent ophthalmology consult. How will the nurse prepare this patient for transport?

★ GLAUCOMA

PATHOPHYSIOLOGY

GLAUCOMA is a group of eye diseases that cause an increase in intraocular pressure and compression of the optic nerve. Most glaucomas are chronic in nature and develop slowly and painlessly over time. The emergency nurse should be familiar with the visual impact of these chronic glaucomas as the patient may have a deficit of peripheral vision that can impact communication methods.

ACUTE ANGLE-CLOSURE GLAUCOMA is a medical emergency that occurs when the intraocular pressure increases rapidly to 30 mm Hg or higher (normal pressure is 8 – 21 mm Hg). Permanent vision loss from compression of the optic nerve can occur in as little as a few hours if not rapidly treated. Additionally, scarring of the trabecular meshwork can lead to chronic forms of glaucoma, and cataracts can develop as latent complications. Acute onset commonly occurs in conjunction with pupil dilation, such as when transitioning from light to dark environments.

The following information is for acute angle-closure glaucoma.

DIAGNOSIS

- abrupt onset of pain
- visual changes: described as blurry, cloudy, or halos of light
- headache
- erythema
- corneal edema with clouding
- fixed pupil, mid-dilated (5 – 6 mm)
- Tono-Pen (increased intraocular pressure)
- fundoscopic exam (pale, cupped optic disc)

TREATMENT AND MANAGEMENT

- topical miotic ophthalmic drops to constrict pupil (pilocarpine)
- topical beta blockers
- topical alpha-adrenergic agents (clonidine)
- IV administration of acetazolamide
- IV administration of mannitol
- immediate ophthalmology referral and consult

QUICK REVIEW QUESTION

4. Two patients arrive at the ED separately complaining of acute onset of eye pain. The first patient, a 35-year-old Asian male, describes pain to his left eye as burning, with onset occurring while he was outside in his yard. Clear tearing and erythema are present. The second patient is a 65-year-old Caucasian female who describes her pain as deep and sharp with onset occurring as she was exiting the matinee show at the local movie theater. Which patient does the nurse recognize as needing emergent medical evaluation?

INFECTIONS

- **CONJUNCTIVITIS** (pink eye) is the inflammation of the thin connective tissue that covers the outer surface of the sclera (bulbar conjunctiva) and lines the inner layers of the eyelids (palpebral conjunctiva).

- □ Diagnosis: burning or itching sensation; increased lacrimation (clear or yellow); erythema of sclera and inner eyelids; edema of palpebra; typically no decrease in visual acuity
- □ Management: warm or cool compress for comfort; topical antibiotics if indicated; topical steroid if severe periorbital edema is present; ophthalmic lubricating solution
- ■ **Uveitis** is the inflammation of any of the structures in the uvea, including the iris (iritis or anterior uveitis), the ciliary body (intermediate uveitis), or the choroid (choroiditis or posterior uveitis).
  - □ Diagnosis: pain described as global aching or tenderness; cilliary spasm; conjunctival erythema; photophobia; vision changes; vitreous floaters; keratitis; Tono-Pen (increased intraocular pressure)
  - □ Management: topical mydriatic ophthalmic drops to dilate the pupil; topical corticosteroids; referral to ophthalmology within 24 hours

QUICK REVIEW QUESTION

5. A 35-year-old female with a known history of HIV is diagnosed in the ED with iritis following an acute onset of erythema, tenderness, and photophobia. Clinically, the left pupil is small and irregular in shape. The patient asks the nurse when her eye will "return to normal." What patient education should the nurse anticipate delivering?

DID YOU KNOW?

Acute iritis may take several weeks to resolve. If left untreated it may result in chronic uveitis, which can lead to secondary formation of cataracts, glaucoma, macular edema, and permanent vision loss.

★

Retinal Artery Occlusion

PATHOPHYSIOLOGY

Retinal artery occlusion occurs when there is a blockage of vascular flow through the retinal arteries, resulting in a lack of oxygen delivery to the nerve cells in the retina. Blockage may occur from thrombi or emboli, and is sometimes referred to as an ocular stroke.

HELPFUL HINT

Patients with risk factors for stroke (e.g., hypertension, A-fib, diabetes) are also at risk for retinal artery occlusion.

DIAGNOSIS

- ■ unilateral, sudden, painless loss of vision
- ■ Tono-Pen (increased intraocular pressure)
- ■ dilated fundoscopic exam
  - □ red fovea (cherry-red spot)
  - □ optic disc pallor and edema

TREATMENT AND MANAGEMENT

- ■ topical beta blockers
- ■ IV acetazolamide
- ■ IV mannitol
- ■ IV methylprednisolone
- ■ ocular massage
- ■ immediate referral to ophthalmology

6. A patient is diagnosed with a central retinal artery occlusion of the right eye after experiencing a sudden loss of sight while outside gardening 60 minutes before arrival. The nurse obtains the following medication list from the patient: metformin 500 mg twice daily, chewable aspirin 81 mg daily, warfarin (Coumadin) 5 mg daily, diltiazem (Cardizem) 60 mg three times daily, cetirizine (Zyrtec) 10 mg daily, metoprolol (Lopressor) 25 mg twice daily, and pravastatin 40 mg daily. What risk factors can the nurse identify based upon the diagnosis and medication history?

RETINAL DETACHMENT ✱

PATHOPHYSIOLOGY

DETACHMENT occurs when the pigmented epithelial layer of the retina separates from the choroid layer (visualize how thin layers of an onion peel can separate from each other) either by tension, trauma, or fluid accumulation between the layers. Vision loss results from lack of available oxygen and deterioration of photoreceptor cells.

DIAGNOSIS

- painless onset of visual changes
- loss of vision is not immediate (unlike retinal artery occlusions)
- reduction in peripheral vision and curtain-like shadow over visual field
- sudden or gradual increase of multiple floaters (wispy spider web-like formations that "float" across the visual field)
- fundoscopic exam to assess for Shafer's sign, vitreous hemorrhage, and scleral depression
- ocular ultrasound

TREATMENT AND MANAGEMENT

- stabilize patient and treat underlying injuries
- bedrest and quiet environment
- immediate referral to ophthalmology

QUICK REVIEW QUESTION

7. A 25-year-old female patient arrives at the ED with complaint of "a curtain" shading her peripheral vision and "hazy strings" floating across her visual field. Onset was yesterday but is becoming progressively worse. Medical history is nonsignificant except for tonsillectomy at age 8. The nurse conducts a visual acuity test and the patient states results are consistent with her baseline sight of 20/100 without glasses. Explain how this patient may be at risk for retinal detachment.

OCULAR TRAUMA

Globe Rupture

PATHOPHYSIOLOGY

A **GLOBAL RUPTURE** (open globe) occurs from a full thickness laceration or tearing of the cornea and sclera. Rupture may occur as the result of blunt trauma, penetrating injury (entry wound without exit), or a perforating injury (entry and exit wounds present). Rupture can also occur post-trauma due to a rapid rise in intraocular pressure.

DID YOU KNOW?

Common sources of ocular trauma include occupational injuries, MVCs, and falls (especially children and the elderly).

DIAGNOSIS

- eccentric or teardrop-shaped pupil
- sunken eye appearance and loss of volume
- gross deformity or misshapen eye
- ocular pain
- subconjunctival hemorrhage
- decreased visual acuity
- edema, erythema, or ecchymosis
- tenting of the sclera or cornea at the site of globe puncture
- ultrasound, X-ray, or CT scan to assess for ocular hemorrhage, muscular or nerve damage, and fractures

TREATMENT AND MANAGEMENT

- maintain bedrest; elevate head of bed 30 degrees
- topical anesthetics
- IV analgesics
- IV antiemetics
- Do NOT:
  - irrigate
  - remove foreign body or penetrating objects
  - measure intraocular pressure
  - use pressure or absorbent dressings
- have patient avoid Valsalva maneuvers, eye manipulation, or extraoccular movements
- keep patient NPO and prep for surgery

QUICK REVIEW QUESTION

8. A 22-year-old male patient arrives at the ED after sustaining injury to his left eye during a bar fight. The eye is edematous, there is visual prolapse of the uvea, and vitreous extrusion is present. The patient exhibits signs of pain and is unable to tolerate visual acuity testing at this time. What nursing interventions does the nurse anticipate?

Hyphema

PATHOPHYSIOLOGY

HYPHEMA is a collection of blood inside the anterior chamber between the cornea and iris. Blood accumulates as a result of a traumatic tear in the vascular structure of the iris or pupil, and it may rise to a level that fully occludes all vision.

Hyphema bleeding differs in appearance from bleeding that is seen with a subconjunctival hemorrhage. Hyphema is dependent; the blood rises in a horizontal fashion in front of the iris as it accumulates, similar to how water levels rise in a closed chamber. A SUBCONJUCTIVAL HEMORRHAGE is painless and occurs from rupture of localized surface vessels in the sclera. A subconjunctival hemorrhage is irregularly shaped, covers the white portion of the eye, and does not result in visual deficit or loss.

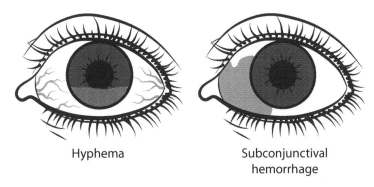

Hyphema   Subconjunctival
                   hemorrhage

Figure 11.2. Hyphema versus Subconjunctival Hemorrhage

DIAGNOSIS

- visible accumulation of blood
- decreased visual acuity
- pain and headache
- Tono-Pen (increased intraocular pressure)

TREATMENT AND MANAGEMENT

- maintain bedrest; elevate head of bed ≥ 45 degrees
- topical corticosteroids
- topical cycloplegics
- topical beta blockers
- topical alpha-adrenergic agents (clonidine)
- IV administration of acetazolamide
- IV administration of mannitol

9. A patient is admitted to the ED with severe inflammation around the right eye. He stated he was hit with a baseball and complains of severe pain, pressure, sensitivity to light, and blurred vision. As the nurse's assessment progresses she notes blood filling the area over the iris under the cornea. What potential diagnosis will this patient receive and what treatment should the nurse anticipate?

Laceration

PATHOPHYSIOLOGY

CORNEAL LACERATIONS extend into the deeper layers of the cornea and are more symptomatic and painful than corneal abrasions. Lacerations are considered partial thickness (closed globe) and do not penetrate the globe structure of the eye.

DIAGNOSIS

- extreme pain or burning sensation
- copious lacrimation
- erythema and edema
- misshapen palpebra, conjunctiva, or external structures
- decrease in visual acuity
- bleeding if vascular structures are involved
- subconjunctival hemorrhage

TREATMENT AND MANAGEMENT

- foreign body removal/irrigation
- topical anesthetic
- topical antibiotics
- topical NSAIDs
- ophthalmic lubricating solution
- suture repair if warranted
- do not use pressure or absorbent dressings
- injectable anesthetics for suture repair; epinephrine will aid in vasoconstriction

QUICK REVIEW QUESTION

10. A patient with a closed globe injury is observed holding a facecloth over the affected eye "for comfort" but has removed the protective eye shield to do so. What complication of introducing external pressure to this eye does the nurse need to monitor for?

ULCERATIVE KERATITIS

PATHOPHYSIOLOGY

ULCERATIVE KERATITIS is characterized by crescent-shaped inflammation of the epithelial layer that progresses to necrosis of the corneal stroma. Ulcers may occur from infectious or noninfectious causes, and they form scar tissue when healing. Without treatment, ulcers may infiltrate deeper structures of the eye, causing secondary uveitis, prolapse of the iris or cilliary body, hypopyon, and endophthalmitis/panophthalmitis.

DIAGNOSIS

- painful pressure, severe pain, or burning sensation
- increased lacrimation
- erythema and edema
- white or cloudy spot on cornea
- sensation of foreign body or grit
- decrease in visual acuity: may be described as blurred, dull, or foggy

TREATMENT AND MANAGEMENT

- nonocclusive eye shield for protection
- topical anesthetic
- topical antibiotics
- topical NSAIDs
- ophthalmic lubricating solution

QUICK REVIEW QUESTION

11. A patient was seen in the ED and diagnosed with a corneal abrasion. The patient returns 6 days later stating that pain has become significantly worse and that the front of his eye appears white in color, impacting his central vision. The patient admits to not completing the course of prescribed antibiotic ophthalmic drops and reinserting his contact lenses the following day. The contact lens remains in the affected eye as the patient was unable to remove it before returning to the ED. How would the nurse explain to the patient how the corneal abrasion progressed to ulcerative keratitis?

ANSWER KEY

1. Determine extent of injury with a slit lamp or Woods lamp exam and use fluorescein staining to assess for presence of corneal abrasions. The cause of the abrasion(s) for this patient is potentially related to use of general anesthesia during recent oral surgery. Anesthesia diminishes the corneal reflexes and decreases basal tear production.

2. Assess pH level with litmus paper or pH indicator strips. (In a pinch, a urinalysis test strip may be used after cutting off test areas above the pH level.) Touch the paper or test strip to the conjunctival fornix. If results are > 7.4, additional irrigation is warranted.

3. Because the patient has an intraocular foreign body, patching the affected eye is appropriate pending exam by ophthalmology. Avoid use of Morgan Lens for irrigation. Apply topical anesthetics and topical NSAIDs for pain management. Apply topical antibiotics for infection prophylaxis.

4. The second patient, the 65-year-old female, has identified risk factors for acute angle-closure glaucoma and presents with an onset of pain that occurred when transitioning from a dark to a light environment. The first patient's symptoms are more consistent with a corneal abrasion or foreign body.

5. Acute iritis can take several weeks to resolve. The patient will require use of topical steroids to decrease inflammation and mydriatic ophthalmic drops to prevent the onset of secondary glaucoma. The mydriatic drops will alter the appearance of the pupil, making it larger. Follow-up with ophthalmology is essential to monitor for secondary complications that can lead to permanent vision loss.

6. This patient appears to have risk factors of diabetes, hypertension, hyperlipidemia, and possible A-fib or vascular disease. These conditions increase risks for development of thrombolytic and atheroembolisms, which can occlude the retinal, cerebral, coronary, or pulmonary arteries.

7. High myopia, or nearsightedness, is a risk factor for retinal detachment. High myopia occurs when the shape of the eye is elongated from front to back, causing tension and stretching of the retinal structure. The stretching can cause a hole or break in the retinal tissue, allowing fluid to enter between the layers, ultimately causing the retina to detach.

8. This patient exhibits signs consistent with an open global rupture. The nurse should initiate NPO status and obtain intravenous access. Pain and nausea should be managed to avoid vagal stimulus. An eye shield may be placed to discourage eye manipulation or movements. Head of bed should be elevated to 30 degrees and bedrest status maintained.

9. Hyphema is a collection of blood inside the anterior space of the eye between the cornea and iris. There will be a resultant increase in intraocular pressure that must be monitored closely and treated if applicable. Bedrest, keeping the head of bed elevated ≥ 45 degrees, and avoiding use of anticoagulant medications and alcohol are standards of care.

10. This patient is at risk for developing an open globe rupture. External pressure can elicit an increase in intraocular pressure, causing strain at the weakest point of the sclera at the insertion point of the extraocular muscles. Eye shield protection is essential during the healing process of corneal lacerations.

11. This patient's symptoms and history are consistent with an infectious corneal ulcer related to contact use. Contact lenses can transfer bacteria to the surface of the eye and essentially trap it under the contact for a prolonged period of time. The patient already had a breach in surface integrity from the preexisting abrasion.

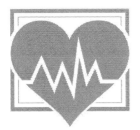

12

ORTHOPEDIC EMERGENCIES

BCEN CONTENT OUTLINE

A. Amputation

B. Compartment syndrome

C. Contusions

D. Costochondritis

E. Foreign bodies

★ F. **FRACTURES/DISLOCATIONS**

G. Inflammatory conditions

H. Joint effusion

★ I. **LOW BACK PAIN**

J. Osteomyelitis

★ K. **STRAINS/SPRAINS**

L. Trauma (e.g., Achilles tendon rupture, blast injuries)

AMPUTATION

PATHOPHYSIOLOGY

AMPUTATION is the total or partial removal of an extremity, including arms, legs, fingers, and toes, either by surgery or trauma or due to illness.

TRAUMATIC AMPUTATIONS may be complete or partial and can occur spontaneously in an uncontrolled (nonsurgical) setting. Particular care needs to be taken to assess for concurrent injury such as fractures, crush injuries, wounds, and vascular compromise.

TREATMENT AND MANAGEMENT (TRAUMATIC AMPUTATION)

- priority: ABCs
- apply direct pressure for bleeding

- IV fluids and blood products as needed
- analgesics
- preserve detached limb
- gently replace attached tissue and maintain normal positioning
- cleanse area with sterile saline solution and cover with thick material
- cover patient to prevent shock

QUICK REVIEW QUESTION

1. A homeless patient arrives in the ED with a complaint of pain in the lower left extremity. The medical history includes untreated diabetes and an infected laceration on the affected leg from a month-old cut. On assessment, the lower leg is pale, cold, and covered in blisters oozing a foul-smelling fluid. What is the nurse's primary concern and what will come next for the patient?

COMPARTMENT SYNDROME

PATHOPHYSIOLOGY

COMPARTMENT SYNDROME is the result of increased intracompartmental pressure, usually as a result of a fracture or crush injury. When the increased pressure in the closed compartment exceeds the pressure of perfusion, blood circulation is impaired, resulting in ischemia of the nerves and muscle tissue. Oxygen deficiency and the buildup of waste produce nerve irritation, resulting in pain and a decrease in sensation. With progression of ischemia, muscles become necrotic, which can lead to rhabdomyolysis, hyperkalemia, and infection if left untreated. Lower legs and arms are the most common areas; however, compartment syndrome can also occur in the abdomen.

DID YOU KNOW?

The most common cause of compartment syndrome is extremity fractures.

SIGNS AND SYMPTOMS

- the 6 P's
  - pain (not proportional to injury and does not respond to opioid medications)
  - paresthesia
  - pallor
  - paralysis
  - pulselessness
  - poikilothermia
- decreased urine output
- hypotension
- tissue tight on palpation
- edema with tight, shiny skin
- intracompartmental pressure > 30 mm Hg or within 20 to 30 mm Hg of MAP

TREATMENT AND MANAGEMENT

- remove casts or dressings to relieve pressure
- analgesics
- IV fluids: maintain urine output > 30 cc/hr
- intracompartmental pressure > 30 mm Hg: prepare patient for fasciotomy
- intracompartmental pressure 10 – 30 mm Hg: monitor pressure and hemodynamic status

QUICK REVIEW QUESTION

2. A patient with an existing Salter-Harris fracture of the right wrist arrives at the ED with acute onset of paresthesia and pain in the distal fingers. The patient states they had a new cast applied yesterday in the outpatient setting. The nurse observes pallor in the extremities and is unable to obtain a radial pulse. What immediate action should the nurse take?

CONTUSIONS

PATHOPHYSIOLOGY

CONTUSIONS appear as ecchymosis and/or hematomas. They are caused by broken blood vessels and the accumulating blood, leakage, or hemorrhage into the soft tissue of the injured area. Most often these injuries are caused by blunt force or mechanical trauma such as a kick, blow, or fall, and occur internally without disrupting the outer skin integrity. Generally, symptoms start to resolve in days. However, serious complications can result from infection, blood clots, calcification, and development of cysts that may require surgery.

DIAGNOSIS

- intact skin
- discoloration (blue, purple, ecchymotic)
- edema
- pain or tenderness
- ultrasound or CT scan if clot is suspected

TREATMENT AND MANAGEMENT

- elevation of contusion
- elastic bandage compress
- cold compress for new injuries at 10-minute intervals; heat for older injuries
- follow up for lump on the bruised area, abnormal pain or bleeding

QUICK REVIEW QUESTION

3. A 10-year-old patient presents to the ED with several small contusions and one large contusion on the thigh following a bicycle wreck. The patient was wearing a helmet and denies hitting her head. What can the nurse implement to reduce the pain and swelling of the larger contusion?

COSTOCHONDRITIS

PATHOPHYSIOLOGY

COSTOCHONDRITIS is the inflammation of the costal cartilage, which joins the ribs to the sternum. It usually affects the fourth, fifth, and sixth ribs. The inflammation causes the chest wall to be tender and painful upon palpation. There is no known definite cause, and the condition will generally resolve without treatment.

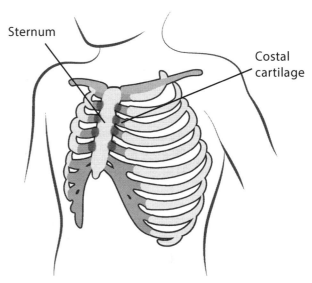

Figure 12.1. Costochondritis

HELPFUL HINT

Idiopathic costochondritis is more common in women, particularly children and teenagers.

SIGNS AND SYMPTOMS

- sharp pain at chest wall; radiating to abdomen or back
- tenderness on palpation of rib joints
- rib pain increases with deep breathing and movement of the trunk
- can cause dyspnea or anxiety

TREATMENT AND MANAGEMENT

- application of heat or ice
- anti-inflammatories
- steroid injection with local anesthetic if anti-inflammatory is ineffective
- rest and avoidance of sports and exercise

4. What clinical findings would lead the nurse to suspect costochondritis in a 13-year-old girl with a complaint of chest pain?

FRACTURES ★

PATHOPHYSIOLOGY

A **FRACTURE** is any break in a bone. **OPEN FRACTURES** include a break in the skin; with a **CLOSED FRACTURE**, the skin is intact. Open fractures create the potential for infection via bacteria entering through the open skin.

Further classifications of fractures are made based on the configuration of the fracture.

- **NON-DISPLACED:** Broken area of the bone remains in alignment; this is the optimal condition for reduction and healing.

- **DISPLACED:** Broken areas of bone are not aligned. It may require manual or surgical reduction including hardware for fixation.

- **TRANSVERSE:** A horizontal break in a straight line across the bone occurs from a force perpendicular to the break.

- **OBLIQUE:** A diagonal break occurs from a force higher or lower than the break.

- **SPIRAL:** A torsion or twisting break around the circumference of the bone is common in sports injuries.

- **COMMINUTED:** The break is fragmented into 3 or more pieces. This is more common in people older than 65 and those with brittle bones.

- **COMPRESSION:** The break is crushed or compressed, creating a wide, flattened appearance. It frequently occurs with crush injuries.

- **SEGMENTAL:** Two or more areas of the bone are fractured, creating a segmented area of "floating" bone.

- **GREENSTICK:** In this type of incomplete break, the bone is not completely separated and bends to one side; it is common in children.

- **AVULSED:** A "chip" fracture displaces small segments of bone from the main bone at the area of tendon/ligament attachment. It results from tension/pulling of the tendons/ligaments away from the bone.

- **TORUS/BUCKLE FRACTURE:** This is an incomplete fracture with bulging of the cortex, common in children.

- **IMPACTED:** The ends of the bone are impacted or "jammed" into each other from forceful impact.

- **SALTER-HARRIS:** This is a growth plate fracture, classified as I – V.

DID YOU KNOW?

Fat embolism syndrome is a condition in which circulating fat emboli cause respiratory, cardiac, and skin symptoms. It is rare, but can occur after fractures of the femur, tibia, or pelvis.

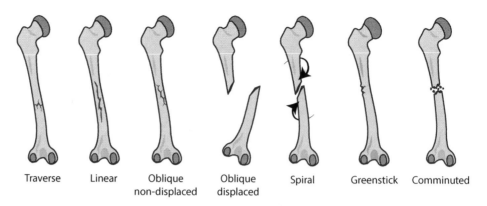

| Traverse | Linear | Oblique non-displaced | Oblique displaced | Spiral | Greenstick | Comminuted |

Figure 12.2. Types of Fractures

DIAGNOSIS

- pain and tenderness increasing with movement
- swelling
- visual or palpated deformity
- crepitus
- abnormal movement or decreased ROM
- inability to bear weight
- contusions or bleeding
- X-ray for injury

TREATMENT AND MANAGEMENT

- analgesics
- cleanse open wounds
- monitor for hemorrhage and hypovolemic shock (due to external or internal blood loss
- reduce (manual or surgical as indicated)
- immobilize
- Splints: non-circumferential, applied for acute care, and allow space for swelling while awaiting orthopedic consult
- Casts: circumferential, more effective with immobilization, and more permanent

HELPFUL HINT

estimated blood loss for fractures:

pelvic fracture: 1.5 – 4.5 L

hip fracture: 1.5 – 2.5 L

femur fracture: 1 – 2 L

humerus fracture: 1 – 2 L

QUICK REVIEW QUESTION

5. A teenage male was admitted to the ED following a fall on outstretched hand (FOOSH) that occurred while skateboarding. The patient denied hitting his head and complains of nausea and pain increasing with movement. The physical assessment findings are tenderness, slight deformity, lateral and medial bruising, and progressive swelling to the affected (left) hand. Radial pulse is strong and palpable and capillary refill time is brisk. No pallor of the extremity is present. What should the nurse do next?

DISLOCATIONS

PATHOPHYSIOLOGY

DISLOCATIONS occur when the two bones of a joint are separated and it no longer functions as a single unit. Deformity of the joint will remain until it is realigned and put back in place. The most common joints dislocated include the shoulder and fingers. However, dislocations of the knees, hips, and elbows can occur.

DIAGNOSIS

- joint noticeably deformed or displaced
- edema
- contusions
- extreme pain
- decreased or no ROM
- X-ray or MRI

TREATMENT AND MANAGEMENT

- analgesics
- reduce or maneuver bones into position with anesthetic
- immobilize joint with splint or sling
- surgery if unable to reduce or nerve, vascular, or ligament damage

QUICK REVIEW QUESTION

6. A woman over the age of 65 is admitted to the ED after falling from a ladder. She reports severe pain and tenderness in her right shoulder and is unable to move it. Following the physical exam, the nurse determines there is a dislocation. What signs and symptoms would the nurse likely have observed on assessment?

INFLAMMATORY CONDITIONS

PATHOPHYSIOLOGY

Inflammatory conditions occur from the immune system attacking the body's own cells or tissues or from accumulation of chemical byproducts causing acute inflammation in the connective tissues. Inflammation causes a thickening of the synovial membrane and leads to irreversible damage to the joint capsule and cartilage from scarring. Both acute and chronic conditions result in pain, erythema, swelling, stiffness.

Common inflammatory conditions include:

- rheumatoid arthritis
- psoriatic arthritis
- osteoarthritis
- ankylosing spondylitis

- scleroderma
- gout
- Sjogren's syndrome
- systemic lupus erythematosus

SIGNS AND SYMPTOMS

- erythema
- pain, edema, stiffness, deformity, and loss of function in joints
- fever or chills
- muscle pain and stiffness

TREATMENT AND MANAGEMENT

- treatment based on disease type, age, health, history, and severity of disease
- treat underlying disease
- topical or oral analgesics (NSAIDs)
- corticosteroids
- discharge teaching: rest, assistive devices

QUICK REVIEW QUESTION

7. A 75-year-old woman arrives at the ED complaining of severe pain in both hands. She has limited income and has not sought prior treatment. She states the pain has increased recently, she is progressively losing function of her hands, and her knees have recently started hurting as well. On assessment the nurse finds the joints in both hands to be reddened, swollen, and disfigured, and the patient's knees slightly swollen. What condition should the patient's symptoms lead the nurse to suspect?

JOINT EFFUSION

PATHOPHYSIOLOGY

JOINT EFFUSION, or a swollen joint, occurs when the normally small amount of fluid in the synovial compartment of a joint increases. The additional fluid can be the result of infection, inflammation (often from an autoimmune condition), or trauma.

DIAGNOSIS

- deep, throbbing pain in joints
- skin warm on palpation
- stiffness and decreased ROM in joints
- edema and erythema around joints

TREATMENT AND MANAGEMENT

- analgesics
- NSAIDs
- steroids
- anti-inflammatory or steroid injections
- disease-modifying anti-rheumatic drugs (DMARDs)
- remove fluid
- colchicine (for gout)
- antibiotics (for infection)

QUICK REVIEW QUESTION

8. A patient with a history of osteoarthritis comes to the ED with complaints of knee pain that is progressively getting worse. The X-ray results show joint effusion. What should the nurse expect to find on the physical assessment?

LOW BACK PAIN ★

PATHOPHYSIOLOGY

LOW BACK PAIN can arise from any of the anatomical structures of the back, including vertebrae, intervertebral discs, spinal nerves, or any of the muscles, tendons, and ligaments found in the lower back. The pain can be classified as either radiating or non-radiating. Pathology of non-radiating lower back pain is typically unknown or idiopathic in nature, but the pathology of radiating lower back pain is usually more apparent.

Causes of lower back pain include:

- sprains and strains: acute injuries to muscles, tendons, or ligaments, often from rapid lifting or twisting motions
- disc hernia, rupture, or degeneration: intervertebral discs bulging, rupturing, or degenerating with age
- cauda equina syndrome: a complication of a ruptured disc in which compression causes an onset of bowel, bladder, and sexual dysfunction that can become permanent if not quickly treated
- compression fractures: weakening and breaking of the vertebrae (often due to osteoporosis)
- radiculopathy: compression, inflammation, or injury of spinal nerve roots
- sciatica: compression of the sciatic nerve that produces radiating pain that travels the nerve path from the buttock through the posterior leg

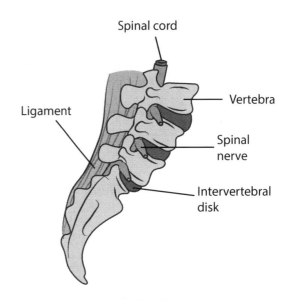

Figure 12.3. Anatomy of the Spine

- spondylolisthesis: occurs when a vertebra of the lower spine slips out of place, pinching a spinal nerve
- spinal stenosis: narrowing of the spinal column that can compress the spinal cord and spinal nerves
- infections: infection of the vertebrae (osteomyelitis), discs (discitis), or sacroiliac joints (sacroiliitis)
- tumors and cysts: rare cause of back pain, but may occur from metastasis of cancer from elsewhere in the body
- other conditions that present with lower back pain as a symptom: kidney stones, abdominal aortic aneurysm, osteoporosis, endometriosis, fibromyalgia

TREATMENT AND MANAGEMENT

- treatment based on injury type and severity
- topical and oral analgesics
- corticosteroids
- muscle relaxers
- nerve block
- lumbar support brace or pillow

QUICK REVIEW QUESTION

9. A retired nurse is admitted to the emergency room with complaints of severe lower back pain. The patient states he has bulging disks; however, the pain has progressed over the past month and now pain has been radiating down his left leg since he lifted a heavy box at home. The nurse's assessment finds tenderness on the lower spine and the patient cannot straight-lift his legs. What is the most likely cause of the current condition?

OSTEOMYELITIS

PATHOPHYSIOLOGY

OSTEOMYELITIS is an infection in the bone that can occur directly (after a traumatic bone injury) or indirectly (via the vascular system or other infected tissues). In children, osteomyelitis is most commonly found in the long bones of the upper and lower extremities, while in adults it is most common in the spine.

HELPFUL HINT
Spreading infection from open wounds (e.g., fractures) are the most common cause of osteomyelitis.

DIAGNOSIS

- may be asymptomatic
- fever or chills
- pain at site of infection
- s/s of local infection (warmth, exudate)
- labs show infection
- bone biopsy to diagnose

TREATMENT AND MANAGEMENT

- debride bone and tissue
- incision and drainage
- long course of IV antibiotics
- surgery may be required for re-vascularization, tissue/bone graft, or removal of medical devices

QUICK REVIEW QUESTION

10. A noncompliant patient with diabetes who has peripheral neuropathy admits to the ED complaining of sudden severe pain on the plantar surface of their right foot. The patient is obese, lives alone, and admits to not doing foot checks. The nurse's assessment finds a temperature of 100.9°F (38.3°C), with vital signs otherwise stable. A foot ulcer is noted to be erythemic surrounding the perimeter of the wound and has a necrotic wound bed with foul-smelling purulent discharge. The nurse believes this patient has osteomyelitis. What is the best test to confirm this diagnosis?

STRAINS AND SPRAINS   ★

PATHOPHYSIOLOGY

Both strains and sprains are very common injuries and share similar signs and symptoms. SPRAINS involve the tearing or stretching of ligaments, whereas STRAINS involve the tearing or stretching of muscle or tendons. Acute strains are from pulling or stretching the muscle abruptly. Chronic strains occur from repeated movements of a muscle.

SIGNS AND SYMPTOMS

- pain
- edema
- sprains: contusion, decreased ROM, hear or feel a pop on incident
- strains: spasms, decreased ability to move muscle
- X-ray to rule out fracture

TREATMENT AND MANAGEMENT

- mild sprains or strains typically treated at home
- ice, compression, and elevation
- analgesics
- immobilization for severe injury

QUICK REVIEW QUESTION

11. A patient arrives at the ED with a complaint of lower back pain occurring when shoveling 6 inches of snow. There is no prior history of back issues and the patient is 25 years old. The nurse determines it is most likely a strain. What brought the nurse to this conclusion?

TRAUMA

Achilles Tendon Rupture

PATHOPHYSIOLOGY

The **ACHILLES TENDON** links the calf muscle to the heel bone. When this tendon is overstretched it may partially or completely tear, resulting in the inability to walk.

SIGNS AND SYMPTOMS

- pain and tenderness
- swelling
- stiffness before activity
- decreased strength
- hearing or feeling a pop on occurrence
- unable to flex foot or push off on toes when walking
- gap felt on palpation of area of rupture
- ultrasound or MRI

TREATMENT AND MANAGEMENT

- ice
- analgesics
- stabilize ankle flexed downward (walking boot or cast)
- may require surgery

QUICK REVIEW QUESTION

12. A patient arrives at the ED unable to walk due to intensifying calf pain. What assessments can the nurse do to confirm a ruptured Achilles tendon?

Blast Injury

PATHOPHYSIOLOGY

BLAST INJURIES result from proximity to an explosion, and the severity of the injury will vary with the type and size of the explosion and its distance from the body. Blast injuries are placed into four categories.

1. **PRIMARY BLAST INJURIES** are caused by the over-pressurization shock wave that results from a high-explosive detonation (e.g., dynamite). Primary blast injuries result in **BAROTRAUMA** (injuries caused by increased air pressure) to hollow gas-filled structures such as the lungs, GI tract, and ear drums.

2. **SECONDARY BLAST INJURIES** occur from flying debris impacting the body and causing blunt or penetrative trauma.

3. **TERTIARY BLAST INJURIES** result from the human body being thrown against a hard surface by the blast of an explosion.

HELPFUL HINT

Blast lung injury (BLI) is a primary injury seen after an explosion and is characterized by respiratory difficulties with no external signs of injury.

4. **QUATERNARY BLAST INJURIES** are any symptoms not categorized as primary, secondary, or tertiary. Often, quaternary blast injuries are existing conditions (e.g., heart disease) that are exacerbated by the explosion.

SIGNS AND SYMPTOMS

- primary injuries
- blast lung injuries (BLI) clinical triad: apnea, hypotension, bradycardia
- ruptured tympanic membrane (possible predictor of BLI)
- secondary and tertiary injuries: lacerations, penetrating injuries, crush injuries, fractures

TREATMENT AND MANAGEMENT

- treatment based upon extent of injury; may include care of traumatic amputation, fractures, burns, or wounds (See above and Ch. 13, "Wound Emergencies," for management of individual conditions.)
- BLI: airway management, likely intubation and ventilation

QUICK REVIEW QUESTION

13. A patient arrives at the ED after an explosion at a fireworks factory. Witnesses stated the patient was placing a wick when the explosion occurred. Assessment findings include second- and third-degree burns to face, neck, bilateral hands, and arms. The patient's blood pressure is 90/76 mm Hg, HR is 42 bpm, and RR is 5 with episodes of apnea. Tympanic membranes are ruptured and a butterfly pattern is seen on X-ray. IV fluids and high-flow oxygen were started on arrival and labs are pending. What should the nurse prepare for next?

ANSWER KEY

1. The patient exhibits signs and symptoms of gangrene associated with the infected laceration, possible sepsis, and untreated diabetes. The nurse should begin preparing the patient for surgery for removal of the affected leg.

2. Remove the cast ASAP, reassess circulation, sensation, movement, and neurovascular status. If compartment syndrome is suspected, prepare for emergent fasciotomy or surgical consult.

3. The nurse should administer an analgesic, elevate the extremity above heart level if possible, and apply ice packs at 10-minute intervals to decrease internal bleeding.

4. Chest pain with tenderness on palpation of the fourth, fifth, and sixth ribs is the classic sign of costochondritis. Myocardial chest pain is less common in young patients.

5. The patient has signs and symptoms consistent with a left wrist fracture. X-rays will be required to assess the extent of injury and bone(s) involved. The nurse should anticipate administering analgesic medication and assisting with orthocasting or splinting of the hand until orthopedic referral can be arranged.

6. Signs and symptoms of dislocation would include reported severe pain, deformity, bruising, decreased or no ROM, and swelling.

7. The nurse should suspect the patient has rheumatoid arthritis. The patient exhibits several physical findings relating to this disease: it is progressive, affects bilateral joints, and causes disfigurement.

8. Findings could include deep, throbbing pain; warm, reddened skin; stiffness; decreased ROM; and swelling.

9. A herniated disk or disks has applied pressure to the spinal nerves, causing shooting pain and the inability to raise her legs. The heavy lifting at home most likely caused the disk to herniate.

10. A bone biopsy is considered the gold standard for diagnosing. The patient will require a surgical procedure to obtain the bone specimen. In the interim, broad-spectrum IV antibiotics should be initiated.

11. The diagnosis is based on the patient's statement of activity when the injury occurred. Risks for strains include lifting heavy objects (snow) and awkward positioning (shoveling).

12. The nurse should ask the patient if they heard or felt a pop when the pain occurred. The nurse should also evaluate the patient's ability to flex the toes downward and assess for swelling, tenderness, and/or a gap on palpation.

13. Patient is exhibiting symptoms of blast lung injury. Intubation will be essential and tracheotomy may be considered if airway damage and swelling prohibits advancement of ET tube.

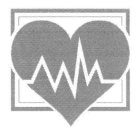

WOUND EMERGENCIES

BCEN CONTENT OUTLINE

TRAUMA ★

Table 13.1. Diagnosis and Management of Trauma Wounds

WOUND	MANAGEMENT
FIRST DEGREE (OR STAGE 1) ABRASIONS minor injuries resulting from superficial damage to the epidermis; bleeding does not occur, but moist serous drainage may be present **SECOND DEGREE (STAGE 2) ABRASIONS** extend into the upper dermal layers; scant bleeding can occur and risk for infection and scarring increases with deeper tissue involvement	• irrigate wound • cleanse area with saline solution or mild soap and water • topical antibiotic • topical anesthetic or ice • cover using clean, moist dressing or nonstick/non-adherent dressing

Table 13.1. Diagnosis and Management of Trauma Wounds (continued)

WOUND	MANAGEMENT
AVULSION full thickness injury in which skin is separated from the body by an external force tearing or pulling the tissue; exposed ligaments, tendons, muscle fibers, and bone may be visible **DEGLOVING INJURY** an avulsion where the skin is completely separated from the underlying structures	• control bleeding • local or topical anesthetic • analgesics • debride wound (remove detached tissues as needed) • irrigate wound with saline solution (avoid application of soap, hydrogen peroxide, or alcohol directly on wound) • cover wound with an absorbent, non-adhering bandage or dressing • compression bandage and ice if needed • antibiotics
FOREIGN BODIES key indicator of a foreign body is inflammation; the timing of the reaction and the amount of inflammation depends on the composition of the foreign body	• remove foreign object(s) and cleanse area thoroughly by irrigating with saline solution
LACERATION a tear of the soft tissue; external lacerations that involve full thickness of the skin layers into the subcutaneous tissue are at high risk for infection due to bacteria or debris from the object causing the injury	• control bleeding • local anesthetic • analgesics • irrigate with normal saline • prepare for closure with suturing, stapling, Dermabond adhesive, or Steri Strips as appropriate • dress wound • ice • antibiotics
INJECTION INJURY Injection of substances (e.g., paint, grease, industrial chemicals) through an almost unseen point of entry via high-pressure equipment; can result in tissue necrosis, compartment syndrome, or contractures	• debride, irrigate, and dress wound • prophylactic antibiotics • surgical consult ASAP • monitor for compartment syndrome
MISSILE INJURY damage from a projectile (e.g., bullet); injury is dependent on the type, trajectory, and velocity of the bullet and on the characteristics of the tissue or organs involved	• remove clothing • primary survey for entry/exit wounds; secondary survey to diagnose all injuries • imaging: CT angiogram, eFAST, X-ray, or MRI • IV fluids or blood products as needed • pressure/tourniquet to bleeding injuries • analgesics • surgical consult

WOUND	MANAGEMENT
PUNCTURE WOUNDS caused by an object entering through soft tissue, resulting in hemorrhage and damage to the skin and underlying tissues; the penetrating object also deposits organisms or foreign bodies into the deeper tissue, increasing the risk for infection	• irrigate wound with saline solution • topical anesthetic or ice • cover using clean, moist dressing or nonstick/non-adherent dressing • antibiotics

QUICK REVIEW QUESTION

1. A patient is treated in the ED following a bicycle accident. The patient has a large area of "road rash" along the right outer leg and across both palms. The wounds present with scant bleeding and serous drainage mixed with copious amounts of dirt and debris. Fractures and vascular injury have been ruled out, and full range of motion is intact. What should the nurse anticipate for wound care for this patient?

INFECTIONS ★

PATHOPHYSIOLOGY

Trauma wounds are at high risk for infection because they are contaminated by debris and microorganisms. Surgical site infections may also require emergency care, particularly if the patient had a preexisting infection or there was spillage from the GI tract during surgery. If not treated properly wound infections prevent proper healing and may lead to complications including cellulitis, endocarditis, septicemia, and osteomyelitis.

DID YOU KNOW?

Wound infection is more likely to occur in patients with diabetes, malnutrition, decreased mobility, impaired circulation, or depressed immune systems.

DIAGNOSIS

■ fever

■ pain, erythema, and edema around wound

■ purulent exudate from wound

■ CBC with differential and cultures to identify infectious organism

TREATMENT AND MANAGEMENT

■ wound care, including drainage, debridement, and appropriate dressings

■ incision and drainage of abscesses

■ topical antibiotics for non-purulent, local infections

■ oral antibiotics for purulent local infections

■ IV antibiotics for systemic infections or high-risk patients

2. A 34-year-old patient presents to the ED with a 4-day-old knife wound on her right palm that occurring while slicing vegetables. Her palm is red and swollen, and the nurse notes purulent discharge from the wound. The patient's vital signs are normal. What intervention should the nurse anticipate?

PRESSURE ULCERS

PATHOPHYSIOLOGY

PRESSURE ULCERS (also known as pressure injuries, decubitus ulcers, or bedsores) are wounds occurring secondary to tissue ischemia. Unrelieved pressure is the most common cause, with the majority of wounds occurring over a bony prominence. Unrelieved pressure compromises the blood flow to the skin and underlying tissue, which deprives the tissue of oxygen and nutrients and also limits waste removal. Pressure ulcers are described as stage 1 through stage 4; they can also be labeled as a deep tissue injury or unstageable (criteria are given below).

DIAGNOSIS

- stage 1: intact skin
  - area of localized erythema in patients with light-pigmented skin; area of localized blue, purple, or dark red hue in patients with dark-pigmented skin
  - non-blanchable
  - pain present as itching or burning sensation
- stage 2: partial-thickness tissue loss
  - dermis exposed; pink wound bed without slough
  - intact or ruptured blisters (serum or serosanguinous filled)
  - pain present as a deeper itching or burning sensation
- stage 3: full thickness; tissue loss up to, but not including, the fascia
  - subcutaneous tissue exposed
  - slough and eschar
  - pain lessened as nerve damage occurs
- stage 4: full-thickness tissue loss extending through the fascia
  - visibly exposed bone, tendons, and muscle
  - slough and eschar
  - pain may not be present because of complete damage to nerve endings and eschar tissue
- unstageable: unable to measure depth because of obscured view (full-thickness skin or tissue loss is covered with slough/eschar)
- deep tissue injury (DTI): injury to subcutaneous tissue under intact skin
  - non-blanching dark red, maroon, or purple discoloration
  - blood-filled blister or separated blister with dark wound bed

TREATMENT AND MANAGEMENT

■ treat per facility policy and stage of wound

■ reduce pressure on affected area

■ analgesics

■ cleanse per wound consult instructions

■ do not remove eschar, rupture blister, or remove top layer of blister if ruptured

■ antibiotics and monitor signs of infection

QUICK REVIEW QUESTION

3. An elderly patient is admitted to the ED from an extended care facility. On assessment the nurse finds a 10 × 10 cm full-thickness wound on the coccyx. Upon further assessment there is undermining and adipose tissue present; however, no bone or tendon is observed. What stage will the nurse assign to this wound?

ANSWER KEY

1. The nurse should identify that the patient has a mix of stage 1 and stage 2 abrasions. The nurse should prepare to irrigate with saline solution or assist the patient in cleansing with mild soap and water. The nurse will apply topical antibiotic ointment if ordered, and cover the wounds with nonstick or moist dressings. Ice can be applied over the dressing to assist with vasoconstriction and pain relief.

2. The patient has a local wound infection with no systemic symptoms. The nurse should expect to irrigate and dress the wound, and the patient will likely be prescribed oral antibiotics.

3. Stage III is defined as full-thickness skin and tissue loss no deeper than adipose tissue. Tunneling and undermining may or may not be present.

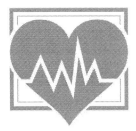

14

ENVIRONMENT

BCEN CONTENT OUTLINE

✳ **A. BURNS**
  B. Chemical exposure (e.g., organophosphates, cleaning agents)
  C. Electrical injuries
  D. Envenomation emergencies (e.g., spiders, snakes, aquatic organisms)
  E. Food poisoning
  F. Parasite and fungal infestations (e.g., giardia, ringworm, scabies)
  G. Radiation exposure
✳ **H. SUBMERSION INJURY**
✳ **I. TEMPERATURE-RELATED EMERGENCIES** (e.g., heat, cold, and systemic)
  J. Vector-borne illnesses
    1. Rabies
    2. Tick-borne illness (e.g., Lyme disease, Rocky Mountain spotted fever)

BURNS ✳

PATHOPHYSIOLOGY

BURNS are trauma to the skin or underlying tissue caused by heat, radiation, electricity, or chemical exposure. The heat causes protein denaturation of the cells that leads to coagulative necrosis, platelet aggregation, and vessel constriction. The damage leaves the dermis open to bacterial infections and fluid loss, possibly leading to hypovolemia and hypothermia.

Burns are classified by depth as first degree, second degree, and third degree.

- **SUPERFICIAL** (first degree): Damage is limited to the epidermis and does not result in blisters (e.g., sunburn).

- **PARTIAL-THICKNESS** (second degree): Damage includes the dermis and epidermis accompanied by severe pain.

- **FULL-THICKNESS** (third degree): All layers of the skin are damaged and there is likely underlying tissue damage. The patient may not feel pain in areas of significant nerve damage.

Burns are described by the **TOTAL BODY SURFACE AREA (TBSA)** involved. TBSA is calculated by assigning a numerical value to the areas that are burned; the rule of 9s is the most commonly used method.

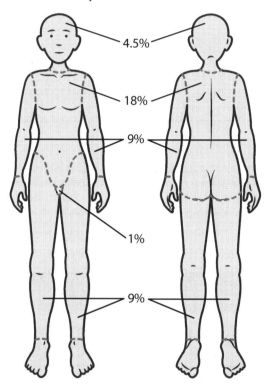

Figure 14.1. Rule of 9s for Calculating Total Body Surface Area (TBSA) of Burns

DIAGNOSIS

- first degree: reddened area that blanches easily with light pressure; pain and swelling

- second degree: white or red; does not blanch; development of vesicles or bullae

- third degree: varying color; no pain or reduced pain (due to nerve damage); no development of vesicles or bullae

- labs to monitor for hypovolemia, electrolyte imbalances, metabolic acidosis, and renal dysfunction

- calculate TBSA (used to correct hypovolemia)
- IV lactated Ringer's per Parkland formula:
  - □ 4 ml × TBSA (%) × body weight (kg)
  - □ Give 50% in first 8 hours; then 50% in next 16 hours.
  - □ Formula time starts at the time the burn happens.
  - □ Expected urine output is 0.5 ml/kg/hr in adults and 0.5 – 1.0 ml/kg/hr in children < 30 kg.
- analgesics
- clean wounds and apply sterile dressing
- topical antibiotic (e.g., silver sulfadiazine)
- escharotomy to remove constricting areas of eschar as needed
- full-thickness burns require hospitalization for excision and grafting

QUICK REVIEW QUESTION

1. A patient presents to the ED with second degree burns on their legs. The nurse establishes that the patient is breathing and has a pulse. What should the nurse prepare to do next?

CHEMICAL EXPOSURE

PATHOPHYSIOLOGY

Chemical exposure can result from inhaling, eating or drinking, or otherwise coming in contact with chemical agents. The injury will depend on the how the patient was exposed, what chemical they were exposed to, and the length of time of the exposure.

In 2012 the hazard communication standard (HCS), which is overseen by OSHA, was revised and now requires all chemical manufacturers, distributers, and importers to provide SAFETY DATA SHEETS (SDS), for all chemical agents. The SDS (formally known as material safety data sheets [MSDS]) for a chemical agent will include information on toxicology, first aid, and exposure control.

DIAGNOSIS

- general s/s: confusion or altered LOC; seizures; dyspnea; nausea and vomiting
- ingestion
  - □ burns, irritation, or redness around the mouth
  - □ breath that smells like chemicals
  - □ abdominal pain

- inhalation
  - □ burning sensation
  - □ increased secretions
  - □ coughing or wheezing
  - □ laryngospasm
- contact
  - □ erythema and edema
  - □ burning or itching
  - □ blisters, hives, or skin discoloration
  - □ pain or numbness of skin
- EGD for ingestion/inhalation
- CXR, spirometry for inhalation

TREATMENT AND MANAGEMENT

- consult poison control and/or SDS
- supportive treatment for s/s
- ingestion
  - □ manage airway
  - □ activated charcoal or antidote if available
  - □ do not administer emetics or gastric lavage
- inhalation
  - □ manage airway
  - □ oxygen as needed
  - □ bronchodilator
  - □ monitor for respiratory dysfunction (e.g., ARDS)
- contact: decontaminate the affected areas: remove patient's clothing and rinse skin with water for 15 – 20 minutes

QUICK REVIEW QUESTION

2. Why is inducing vomiting or gastric lavage contraindicated when a patient has swallowed a chemical?

ELECTRICAL INJURIES

PATHOPHYSIOLOGY

Generated electrical energy causes external and internal injury from the electrical current running through the body. Injuries will vary depending on the intensity of the current, voltage, resistance, the length of time exposed, entry and exit locations, and the tissue and organs affected by the electrical current. Generated electrical injury can result in skin burns, damage to internal organs or tissue, respiratory arrest, or cardiac arrhythmias/arrest.

DID YOU KNOW?

Common complications of lightning strikes include keraunoparalysis, cardiac arrest, and neurological symptoms. Lightning strikes do not usually cause burns, rhabdomyolysis, or internal organ or tissue damage.

DIAGNOSIS

- burns at the entry and exit points with a clean line of demarcation
- involuntary muscular contractions
- dyspnea
- seizures, confusion, or loss of consciousness
- paralysis
- dysrhythmias
- s/s of rhabdomyolysis or compartment syndrome in severe cases

HELPFUL HINT

In patients with electrical injuries, subcutaneous or deeper tissue damage is often greater than the areas indicated by the line of demarcation.

TREATMENT AND MANAGEMENT

- priority: ABCs
- head-to-toe assessment for injuries secondary to falls
- IV fluids
  - standard burn fluid-resuscitation protocols are not used as there is usually more damage than is seen on surface burns
  - IV fluid treatment goal is to maintain urine output of 75 – 100 ml/hr
- analgesics
- monitor cardiac and kidney function

QUICK REVIEW QUESTION

3. A conscious patient comes into the ED and states that he touched a live electrical wire. He has a small injury on his left hand and a small exit injury on the bottom of his left foot, but reports he feels no other symptoms. Why would the nurse proceed with a full electrical injury workup?

ENVENOMATION EMERGENCIES

PATHOPHYSIOLOGY

Most animal bites or stings do not require emergency care and can be managed with OTC analgesics. However, emergent care may be required for exposure to lethal venom or for anaphylaxis. (See Ch. 9, "Medical Emergencies," for detailed information on anaphylactic shock.)

DID YOU KNOW?

Coral snake venom contains a neurotoxin that can cause weakness, paralysis, and respiratory arrest. All patients with coral snake bites should be monitored for at least 12 hours.

Table 14.1. Diagnosis and Management of Envenomation Emergencies

ANIMAL	SIGNS AND SYMPTOMS	TREATMENT AND MANAGEMENT
Snake	• varies depending on snake species • general s/s: nausea and vomiting, tachycardia, diaphoresis • coagulation abnormalities • weakness and lethargy • confusion	• ABCs • antivenom • supportive treatment for s/s

ANIMAL	SIGNS AND SYMPTOMS	TREATMENT AND MANAGEMENT
Spider	• brown spider bites: delayed pain; ecchymosis and erythema; central blood-filled lesion that ruptures, leaving an ulcer • widow spider bites: immediate pain; muscle cramping and weakness; diaphoresis; hypertension; tachycardia	• wound care • analgesics • excision of brown spider bite • opioids and benzodiazepines for symptomatic widow bites • antivenom for widow bites only in patients at high risk for severe systemic response
Scorpion	• immediate pain • possible numbness or stinging • muscular spasms or weakness • restlessness or anxiety • tachycardia • hypertension • increased respiration	• supportive treatment for s/s • antivenom only for patients with severe symptoms
Bee, Wasp, Hornet, or Fire Ant	• immediate pain, burning, and itching • erythema and edema	• remove stinger if still in place • ice, antihistamines, or NSAIDs for pain

QUICK REVIEW QUESTION

4. Why is compression of the area of most bites contraindicated?

FOOD POISONING

PATHOPHYSIOLOGY

FOOD POISONING is an acute infection in the GI system cause by the ingestion of infectious organisms or noninfectious substances. The organism or substance enters through the mouth and produces a toxin or irritant that causes mild to severe acute gastroenteritis in the small intestine. The CDC identifies *Norovirus*, *Salmonella*, *Clostridium perfringens*, *Campylobacter*, and *Staphylococcus aureus* as the top five infectious foodborne agents.

DIAGNOSIS

- onset of symptoms 6 – 24 hours after ingestion
- watery diarrhea
- nausea and vomiting
- abdominal pain and cramping
- chills and/or fever
- generalized weakness and fatigue
- stool culture positive for presence of bacteria, toxins, endotoxins, or parasites

■ supportive treatment: oral fluids, IV fluids, and electrolytes as needed

QUICK REVIEW QUESTION

5. A patient is being discharged with a diagnosis of food poisoning. The patient asks if she can get a prescription or take something OTC to stop the diarrhea. What instructions should the nurse provide?

PARASITE AND FUNGAL INFESTATIONS

■ **GIARDIASIS** is the common name for the parasitic infection cause by *Giardia lamblia*, a flagellated protozoan that attaches itself to the mucosa of the small intestine. The infection disturbs the normal flora in the GI tract, leading to GI upset.

   ☐ Diagnosis: mostly asymptomatic; watery stools; abdominal cramping and pain; flatulence; weight loss; positive enzyme immunoassay or presence of parasite and spores

   ☐ Management: supportive treatment for symptoms; antibiotic/anti-parasite (metronidazole, nitazoxanide)

■ **RINGWORM** is a superficial fungal infection (not actually caused by worms) that only affects the skin. Symptoms and management vary based on the area of infection.

   ☐ **TINEA CAPITIS**: scaling and erythematous patches on the scalp; oral griseofulvin for 6 weeks; shampoo hair 2 – 3 times with ketoconazole (Nizoral) or selenium sulfide shampoo

   ☐ **TINEA CORPORIS**: characteristic bull's-eye–shaped pink or red skin lesion on trunk or extremities; topical antifungal cream or oral griseofulvin or terbinafine

   ☐ **TINEA PEDIS** (athlete's foot): scaling in between toes or on soles of both feet; vinegar-and-water soak or griseofulvin or terbinafine

   ☐ **TINEA CRURIS**: small red scaling patches in groin area; topical antifungal cream or oral griseofulvin or terbinafine

   ☐ **TINEA UNGUIUM**: thick nail beds that crumble easily; itraconazole or terbinafine

SCABIES is an infection of the skin cause by a mite, *Sarcoptes scabiei*.

   ☐ Diagnosis: red, itchy area on the skin that looks like a pinhole; usually seen between fingers, axillary folds, and the waistband area

   ☐ Management: contact precautions; bag clothing and bed linens; provide new clothes and linens; patient washed with warm soapy water; topical scabicide (left on for 12 – 24 hours); oral ivermectin if topical treatment is not effective

QUICK REVIEW QUESTION

6. A 23-year-old woman presents to the ED with diarrhea and receives a diagnosis of giardiasis. What medication will the patient likely be prescribed?

RADIATION EXPOSURE

PATHOPHYSIOLOGY

RADIATION is high-energy waves or particles that can damage human cells. Radiation is classified as either IONIZING—which damages tissue—or NON-IONIZING. Sources of ionizing radiation include X-rays and radioactive substances (e.g., uranium). Radiation exposure is measured in units called GRAYS (Gy); 1 gray is equal to 1 joule of radiation per kilogram.

Radiation results in tissue damage that can be local (such as burns) or systemic. The degree of tissue injury resulting from radiation exposure depends on several factors, including the dose of radiation, the length of exposure, the type of radiation, and the area and amount of the body that was exposed.

- cutaneous radiation injury: damage to the skin caused by acute exposure to radiation

- focal radiation injury: damage to specific tissues or organs caused by acute, focused exposure to radiation (usually seen in patients undergoing radiation therapy)

- acute radiation syndromes (ARS): result of intense exposure of the whole body to radiation that causes a characteristic set of hematopoietic, GI, and cerebrovascular symptoms

Diagnosis is made based on a history of exposure to radiation, lymphocyte count, and signs and symptoms.

TREATMENT AND MANAGEMENT

- minimize health care worker exposure and be mindful of radiation contamination

- trauma to be treated before radiation poisoning

- decontaminate patient

- supportive treatment for s/s

QUICK REVIEW QUESTION

7. Arriving EMS personnel alert the ED nurse that the patient has been exposed to radiation. What should the ED nurse plan as the first intervention for the patient?

SUBMERSION INJURY

PATHOPHYSIOLOGY

A SUBMERSION INJURY is a respiratory injury or impairment that occurs as a result of being submerged in liquid. The respiratory impairment resulting from submersion leads to hypoxemia, which in turn can lead to organ failure, most notably in the lungs, heart, and brain.

These injuries were previously known as "wet drowning" when water was aspirated or "dry drowning" when the patient had a laryngospasm but did not ingest or aspirate water. The term "near drowning" is another term that is no longer commonly used. Submersion injuries are now classified as NONFATAL or FATAL.

HELPFUL HINT

Signs and symptoms of submersion injury are not necessarily immediate; some respiratory damage may take up to 6 hours to produce symptoms.

DIAGNOSIS

- patient found in or near water
- vomiting
- wheezing
- change in LOC
- s/s of respiratory failure
- ABG shows metabolic acidosis

TREATMENT AND MANAGEMENT

- CPR if needed
- priority: treatment of hypoxemia
  - ☐ start patient on 100% oxygen; titrate down based on serial ABG results
  - ☐ intubation and mechanical ventilation may be needed
- nebulized bronchodilators to relieve bronchospasms or wheezing

QUICK REVIEW QUESTION

8. A patient who was found floating in a body of water is admitted to the ED. The patient is currently on 100% O_2 and the current PaO_2 is 45%. What procedure should the nurse prepare for?

COLD-RELATED EMERGENCIES ★

Hypothermia

PATHOPHYSIOLOGY

HYPOTHERMIA occurs when core body temperature drops below 35°C (95°F), causing a reduction in metabolic rate and in respiratory, cardiac, and neurological functions. When body temperature drops below 30°C (86°F), thermoregulation ceases.

During hypothermia, diuresis and systemic fluid leakage into the interstitial space can lead to hypovolemia. Vasoconstriction due to the cold can mask this hypovolemia. When the patient is rewarmed and the vessels dilate, the patient will go into shock or cardiac arrest if the fluid volume is not replaced.

DIAGNOSIS

- mild hypothermia: 32 – 35°C (90 – 95°F)
- moderate hypothermia: 28 – 32°C (82 – 90°F)
- severe hypothermia: < 28°C (82°F)

- intense shivering that lasts until core body temperature drops below 31°C (87.8°F)

- lethargy, clumsiness, confusion, agitation, or hallucinations

- hypotension

- decreased cardiac function
  - □ initial bradycardia and slow A-fib, then V-fib or asystole
  - □ ECG: will read as injury due to myocardial infarction, but will show a J wave or Osborn wave

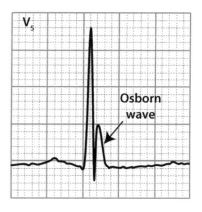

Figure 14.2. Osborn or J Wave

TREATMENT AND MANAGEMENT

- first line: prevent further heat loss by removing wet/cold clothing and insulating patient

- mild hypothermia: passively rewarm patients at a rate of 1°C per hour with an insulated blanket and warmed fluids

- severe hypothermia: active core warming
  - □ inhalation: oxygen at 40°C – 45°C (104°F – 113°F) delivered via oxygen mask or ET tube
  - □ infusion: IV fluids or blood products at 40°C – 42°C (104°F – 107.6°F)
  - □ lavage: closed thoracic lavage through 2 thoracic tubes at 40°C – 45°C (104°F – 113°F)
  - □ Extracorporeal Core Rewarming (ECR) is not often performed as it requires a specialist and prearranged protocol.

- fluid resuscitation: 1 – 2 L (for adults) or 20 ml/kg (for pediatrics) of 0.9% saline solution heated to 40°C – 42°C (104°F – 107.6°F) via IV

- CPR for V-fib or asystole: defibrillation once body temperature > 30°C (86°F)

QUICK REVIEW QUESTION

9.   A patient is admitted to the ED. The patient fell through ice and was submerged in the water for 20 minutes. The patient is unresponsive and has been intubated. How would the nurse prepare oxygen for administration?

Local Cold-Related Emergencies

- **FROSTBITE** is injury to the dermis and underlying tissue due to cold. The exposure to cold leads to cellular damage, impairment of the vascular system, and an inflammatory response.
  - □ Symptoms (early stage): cold and white skin; numbness, tingling, or throbbing in affected area

- □ Symptoms (mild stage): skin hard or frozen to the touch; skin red and blistered when warmed and thawed
- □ Symptoms (severe stage): blue, blotchy, or white skin; black necrotic areas; blood-filled blisters as skin warms; damage to underlying tissue

- ■ **IMMERSION FOOT** is an injury that results from prolonged exposure to a cold and wet environment of a limb that had little or no mobility. The limb will be numb, cold, pale, clammy, and swollen. Severe cases may present with ulcers, eschar, or muscle atrophy.

- ■ Management of frostbite and immersion foot
  - □ rewarm affected area until it is red in color: warm water, heated to 104°F – 108°F (40°C – 42°C), in a basin or bath
  - □ analgesics (pain during rewarming may be severe)
  - □ wound care as necessary, including debridement

- ■ **CHILBLAINS** is an inflammatory response that occurs in the skin and small blood vessels after repeated exposure to cold but not freezing temperatures. It is most common in women, underweight patients, and patients with Raynaud's disease.
  - □ Symptoms: red or purple bumps on the skin that can be painful or swollen; complaints of itchy feeling; blistering or ulceration (severe case)
  - □ Management: passive rewarming of affected area; topical corticosteroids; daily nifedipine for recurrent chilblains

HELPFUL HINT

Do not use hot water or heating pads to manage cold injuries: nerve damage may prevent patients from perceiving burns. Rubbing or massaging should also be avoided because they may cause further damage to tissue.

QUICK REVIEW QUESTION

10. A patient presents to the ED complaining of both hands being numb. The nurse observes that the patient's hands are blue and establishes that the patient has been outside without gloves for several hours. What intervention should the nurse prepare for?

HEAT-RELATED INJURIES ★

- ■ **HEAT CRAMPS** (exercise-associated muscle cramps) occur when exercise or physical exertion leads to a profuse loss of fluids and sodium through sweating. The resulting hyponatremia causes muscle cramps.
  - □ Diagnosis: sudden onset of severe spasmodic muscle cramps in extremities; may progress to carpopedal spasms, which can incapacitate the hands or the feet
  - □ Management: keep patient cool; oral fluids (solution of 1 L of water with 10 g of sodium or commercial sports drinks); IV fluids if patient cannot tolerate fluids by mouth (1 – 2 L of 0.9% saline solution); stretch the affected muscle (firm, passive stretching)

- ■ **HEAT EXHAUSTION** occurs when the body is exposed to high temperatures, leading to dehydration. It is not a result of deficits in thermoregulation or the central nervous system.

- Diagnosis: temperature elevated but < 104°F (40°C); diaphoresis; dizziness and weakness; tachycardia; hypertension; headache; nausea and vomiting; syncope

- Management: cool with ice packs; oral fluids (solution of 1 L of water with 10 g of sodium or commercial sports drinks); IV fluids if patient cannot tolerate fluids by mouth (1 – 2 L of 0.9% saline solution)

■ **HEAT STROKE** (classic or exertional) results when the compensatory measures for ridding the body of excess heat fail, leading to an increased core temperature. Complications can include rhabdomyolysis, DIC, and acute kidney injury.

- Diagnosis: temperature > 104°F (40°C); tachycardia and tachypnea; confusion or delirium; seizures; labs show organ dysfunction

- Management: cool rapidly with ice bath or ice packs to 102°F (38.9°C); aggressive fluid resuscitation; electrolytes as needed; management of complications (e.g., platelets, benzodiazepines)

HELPFUL HINT
Antipyretics are not effective at reducing temperature during heat exhaustion/stroke and may worsen organ dysfunction.

QUICK REVIEW QUESTION

11. A 16-year-old male athlete collapsed during practice and was brought to the ED. His vital signs are as follows:

temperature	105.5°F
HR	120 bpm
RR	22 breaths per minute
BP	95/62 mm Hg

What priority intervention should the nurse anticipate?

VECTOR-BORNE ILLNESSES

■ **LYME DISEASE** is a bacterial infection transmitted through tick bites. Within 3 – 30 days the bacteria will either enter the lymphatic system and cause adenopathy or will continue to circulate in the bloodstream and travel to organs or other skin sites.

- Diagnosis: erythema migrans (first stage); flu-like symptoms (second stage); positive acute and convalescent serologic testing (ELISA confirmed by Western blot)

- Management: oral or IV antibiotics (amoxicillin, doxycycline, ceftriaxone); supportive treatment for symptoms

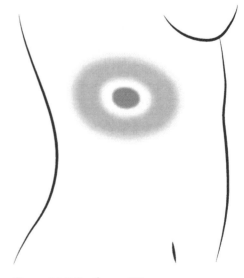

Figure 14.3. Erythema Migrans

- **Rabies** is a virus that causes encephalitis. It is carried in the saliva of infected animals and is transmitted during animal bites.
  - ☐ Diagnosis: fatigue; fever; headache; confusion; agitation; hallucinations; insomnia; excessive salivation; hydrophobia; ascending paralysis; positive fluorescence antibody test from biopsy of skin near the nape of neck
  - ☐ Management: clean wound with soap and water or BZK wipes; rabies vaccine and rabies immune globulin (1.0 ml IM on days 0, 3, 7, and 14); once rabies has advanced, there is no curative treatment
- **Rocky Mountain spotted fever** is an infection caused by *Rickettsia* bacteria, which are carried by hard-shelled ticks. Bacteria lodge in small blood vessels, which become blocked with thrombi, producing vasculitis throughout the body.
  - ☐ Diagnosis: fever, chills, headache, and muscle pain; rash (starts pink and macular, then darkens and becomes maculopapular); positive fluorescent antibody staining in skin biopsy from rash areas; positive PCR
  - ☐ Management: antibiotics (doxycycline); oral or IV chloramphenicol if doxycycline is ineffective; supportive treatment for symptoms

Quick Review Question

12. What type of rash on the skin should prompt the nurse to suspect a patient has Lyme disease? What other tests need to be performed to confirm the diagnosis of Lyme disease?

ANSWER KEY

1. The nurse should prepare to establish IV access; 18 is the preferred needle gauge, with 2 accesses if possible.

2. Vomiting or gastric lavage is contraindicated when a patient swallows a chemical because it may cause further damage to the upper airway or throat and mouth.

3. The total amount of internal damage cannot be judged based on external damage. Internal injury or organ dysfunction could still be present even when the patient has little to no external damage and is presenting asymptomatically.

4. Compression may keep the poison in the area, increasing localized damage.

5. Antidiarrheals are contraindicated for patients who have been positively diagnosed with food poisoning. The diarrhea is the body's way of expelling the infectious organism or noninfectious substance. If the diarrhea is stopped, the offending substance will remain in the small intestine, and the patient will remain sick and may worsen.

6. The patient will likely be prescribed either metronidazole or tinidazole.

7. The first nursing intervention/concern is decontamination. The nurse should remove the patient's clothing and wash their skin, hair, and wounds.

8. The nurse should prepare the patient to be intubated.

9. The oxygen needs to be heated to 40°C – 45°C (104°F – 113°F) before being administered to this patient.

10. The nurse should gather materials to immerse the patient's hands in warm water.

11. The patient is hyperthermic and does not require immediate respiratory intervention. The priority intervention will be rapid cooling with an ice bath or ice packs.

12. Lyme disease presents with a red bull's-eye–shaped rash. Other rashes can be similar in appearance to erythema migrans, so a positive ELISA test is needed to confirm Lyme disease.

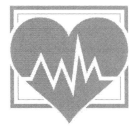

15

TOXICOLOGY

BCEN CONTENT OUTLINE

A. Acids and alkalis

B. Carbon monoxide

C. Cyanide

D. Drug interactions (including alternative therapies)

✱ **E. OVERDOSE AND INGESTIONS**

F. Substance abuse

✱ **G. WITHDRAWAL SYNDROME**

ACIDS AND ALKALIS

PATHOPHYSIOLOGY

ACIDS are compounds that release hydrogen ions and taste sour; **ALKALIS** are compounds that accept hydrogen ions and are slippery or soapy. On the pH scale (1 to 14), acids have a value lower than 7, alkalis have a value greater than 7, and 7 is neutral. Ingestion of acids and alkalis is most common in young children. Ingestion in adults is usually linked to severe mental illness or suicidal behaviors.

- Common household acids: swimming pool and toilet cleaners, battery acid, anti-rust cleaners

- Common household alkalis: common bleach, drain cleaner

Ingestion of acids usually causes injuries to the upper respiratory tract as the pain and sour taste prompt gagging or spitting, which may lead to aspiration. The acid may also cause coagulative necrosis in the stomach. Alkali ingestion will cause liquefactive necrosis in the esophagus and will continue to cause damage until it has been neutralized.

DIAGNOSIS

- drooling
- dysphagia
- excessive thirst
- visible oral burns
- GI pain
- emesis (can appear brown)
- bleeding in mouth, throat, or stomach
- s/s of esophageal perforation
- stridor or dyspnea
- upper GI endoscopy to evaluate damage

TREATMENT AND MANAGEMENT

HELPFUL HINT

An endoscopy is usually performed on asymptomatic patients if they have ingested acids or alkalis to assess for damage in the GI tract.

- manage airway; intubation for patients with severe oropharyngeal edema or necrosis
- supportive care for symptoms: analgesics, IV fluids
- contraindicated treatments include
  - gastric emptying by emesis
  - activated charcoal
  - neutralizing agents
  - gastric lavage
  - nasogastric tube
- immediate surgery for perforation or necrosis

QUICK REVIEW QUESTION

1. A 15-year-old patient is brought to the ED by her mother, who states that the patient mistook a bottle of ammonia for lemonade and drank it. The mother is very upset that the emergency room staff is not trying to make the patient throw it back up to get it out of her system. How do you explain this action to the patient's mother?

CARBON MONOXIDE

PATHOPHYSIOLOGY

DID YOU KNOW?

Pulse oximeters do not differentiate between oxyhemoglobin and carboxyhemoglobin, so patients with CO poisoning will often have normal pulse oximetry readings.

Carbon monoxide (CO) displaces oxygen from hemoglobin, which prevents the transport and utilization of oxygen throughout the body. Mild **CO POISONING** can be resolved in the ED; severe CO poisoning can lead to myocardial ischemia, dysrhythmias, pulmonary edema, and coma. Sources of CO include smoke from fires, malfunctioning heaters and generators, and motor vehicle exhaust. CO poisoning and cyanide poisoning often occur together.

SIGNS AND SYMPTOMS

- headache
- altered LOC or confusion
- dizziness
- visual disturbances
- dyspnea on exertion
- nausea and vomiting
- muscle weakness and cramps
- syncope, seizure, or coma

TREATMENT AND MANAGEMENT

- 100% oxygen through non-rebreather
- hyperbaric oxygen may be used to treat patients with
  - ☐ carboxyhemoglobin level greater than 25%
  - ☐ cardiopulmonary complications
  - ☐ loss of consciousness
  - ☐ severe metabolic acidosis

QUICK REVIEW QUESTION

2. A patient in the ED is diagnosed with carbon monoxide (CO) poisoning. The patient states that she had carbon monoxide monitors installed with the smoke detectors throughout her house, so this diagnosis can't be right. What education can the nurse provide to the patient regarding proper carbon monoxide detector placement?

CYANIDE

PATHOPHYSIOLOGY

Cyanide interferes with the production of ATP in mitochondria. **CYANIDE POISONING** is rare but usually fatal without medical intervention. Sources of cyanide include smoke from fires, medications (e.g., sodium nitroprusside), and pits/seeds from the family Rosaceae (which includes bitter almonds, apricots, peaches, and apples).

SIGNS AND SYMPTOMS

- bitter almond smell on breath
- anxiety or agitation
- headache
- confusion
- bloody emesis
- diarrhea

- flushed, red skin
- tachycardia and tachypnea
- hypertension

TREATMENT AND MANAGEMENT

- decontaminate patient
- 100% oxygen through a non-rebreather; intubation usually required
- IV fluids
- activated charcoal if airway is not compromised
- cyanide antidotes include: hydroxocobalamin, amyl nitrite, sodium nitrite, and sodium thiosulfate

QUICK REVIEW QUESTION

3. A patient presents to the ED with nonspecific symptoms, including confusion, headache, and vomiting. What situations in a patient's history should alert the ED nurse to the possibility of cyanide poisoning?

OVERDOSE AND INGESTION

Toxidromes

- **TOXIDROMES** are groups of signs and symptoms present in patients who have large amounts of toxins or poisons in the body. General signs and symptoms are given below, but these may vary based on the specific drug (or combination of drugs) ingested.

Table 15.1 Signs and Symptoms of Toxidromes

TOXIDROME	HR	BP	RR	TEMP	BOWEL SOUNDS	PUPILS	SKIN	MENTAL STATUS
ANTICHOLINERGIC	↑	↑	—	↑	↓	↑	dry	agitated and delirious
CHOLINERGIC	—	—	—	—	↑	↓	moist	—
HALLUCINOGENIC	↑	↑	↑	—	↑	↑	—	disoriented
SYMPATHOMIMETIC	↑	↑	↑	↑	↑	↑	moist	agitated and delirious
SEDATIVE-HYPNOTIC	↓	↓	↓	↓	↓	—	dry	lethargic and confused

- Anticholinergic toxidrome
  - □ Substances: antihistamines, antipsychotics, tricyclic antidepressants (TCA), scopolamine, atropine, Atropa belladonna (deadly nightshade)

- Management: GI decontamination with activated charcoal; supportive treatment for symptoms; physostigmine (not for TCA overdose)
- Cholinergic toxidrome
  - Substances: anticholinesterase, insecticides and pesticides, nerve agents (e.g., sarin)
  - Management: oxygen and likely intubation; atropine; oximes (e.g., pralidoxime)
- Hallucinogenic toxidrome
  - Substances: LSD, psilocybin ("magic mushrooms"), mescaline, DMT, salvia divinorum, dextromethorphan (DXM), PCP
  - Management: supportive treatment for symptoms
- Sympathomimetic toxidrome
  - Substances: cocaine, amphetamines, methamphetamines, hallucinogenic amphetamines (MDMA, MDA), khat and related substances (methcathinone, "bath salts"), cold medications, diet supplements containing ephedrine
  - Management: supportive treatment for symptoms
- Sedative-hypnotic toxidrome
  - Substances: benzodiazepines, barbiturates, antipsychotics, zolpidem (Ambien), clonidine, GHB
  - Management: flumazenil (for benzodiazepine overdose); supportive treatment for symptoms

QUICK REVIEW QUESTION

4. A 68-year-old patient is brought to the ED with delirium and hyperthermia. The patient's wife brings his medications, which include tiotropium (Spiriva) for COPD and transdermal scopolamine for nausea. What intervention should the nurse anticipate?

Managing Overdoses

SUBSTANCE	SIGNS AND SYMPTOMS	TREATMENT AND MANAGEMENT
Opioid	respiratory depression, shallow breathing, pinpoint pupils, cyanosis, bradycardia, emesis or gurgling, inability to be aroused	naltrexone, ET tube, mechanical ventilation
Acetaminophen	gastroenteritis, renal failure, pancreatitis, hepatotoxicity leading to multiple organ failure	N-acetylcysteine, activated charcoal
Salicylate	nausea and emesis; tinnitus; fever; confusion; seizures; rhabdomyolysis; acute renal failure; hyperventilation and respiratory alkalosis (early), hypoventilation and respiratory acidosis (late), respiratory failure; hyperactivity that can turn into lethargy	activated charcoal, alkaline diuresis with extra KCl, ET tube, mechanical ventilation

Table 15.2. Managing Overdose

HELPFUL HINT
Presentation of cholinergic overdose:
DUMBELS
Diarrhea
Urination
Miosis
Bronchorrhea, bradycardia, bronchoconstriction
Emesis
Lacrimation
Salivation

DID YOU KNOW?
The Rumack-Matthew nomogram is used to predict hepatic toxicity following acetaminophen overdoses.

Table 15.2. Managing Overdose (continued)

SUBSTANCE	SIGNS AND SYMPTOMS	TREATMENT AND MANAGEMENT
Calcium channel blockers	hyperglycemia, hypotension, bradycardia, reflexive tachycardia, peripheral edema, heart block	high-dose insulin, vasopressors, inotrope
Beta blockers	cardiac: bradycardia, hypotension, bronchospasms, prolonged Q–T interval, prolonged QRS complex, ventricular dysrhythmias, AV block GI: esophageal spasms, hyperkalemia, hypoglycemia	glucagon, dopamine, norepinephrine, ipratropium for patients with esophageal spasms
Digitalis	nausea, emesis, abdominal pain, headache, dizziness, confusion, delirium, blurred vision, halo vision, bradycardia, tachydysrythmias (paroxysmal atrial tachycardia with block most common)	digoxin immune fab, potassium supplementation, atropine in case of AV block or severe bradycardia, lidocaine or phenytoin to prevent cardioversion
Heavy metals	altered LOC, fatigue, muscle and joint pain, hypertension, constipation, nausea and emesis, renal failure, numbness and pain in extremities, anemia, dark eye circles, jaundice, rash, itching, hearing loss, insomnia, depression, mood swings Severe lead toxicity will lead to wrist drop, encephalopathy, colic, and Burton's line (blue-black line on the gums). Mercury poisoning can lead to "mad hatter disease," with signs and symptoms including slurred speech, irritability, and depression.	chelation therapy, dialysis
Iron	stage 1: GI upset, nausea, emesis, pain stage 2 (latent phase): milder GI upset stage 3: shock and metabolic acidosis, dehydration, lactic acid stage 4: hepatotoxicity, necrosis stage 5: bowel obstruction from GI healing leading to scarring	deferoxamine mesylate (DFO) for acute iron toxicity, intermittent phlebotomy for chronic iron toxicity from hemochromatosis
Oral hypoglycemic	mild: dizziness, lightheadedness, nausea severe: altered LOC, CNS depression, seizures, coma, hypokalemia, hypomagnesemia	sulfonylurea supplemented with octreotide if needed for GI symptoms, IV dextrose bolus followed by dextrose 10% continuous infusion
Warfarin	bloody, red, or black tarry stool; pink, red, or dark urine; spitting or coughing up blood; "coffee ground" emesis; hemorrhage	vitamin K

5. A patient presents in the ED with constricted pupils, slow and shallow breathing, confusion, and blue-toned skin. Based on the scene, EMS suspects an opioid overdose. What is the nursing priority for this patient?

ACUTE SUBSTANCE WITHDRAWAL ★

Alcohol Withdrawal

PATHOPHYSIOLOGY

ALCOHOL is a central nervous system depressant that directly binds to gamma-aminobutyric acid (GABA) receptors and inhibits glutamate-induced excitation. Chronic alcohol use alters the sensitivity of these receptors; when alcohol use is stopped, the result is hyperactivity in the central nervous system. Alcohol withdrawal can be fatal.

Chronic alcohol use inhibits the absorption of nutrients, including thiamine and folic acid. Consequently, patients admitted with symptoms of alcohol withdrawal are also at risk for disorders related to vitamin deficiency, including Wernicke's encephalopathy and megaloblastic anemia.

SIGNS AND SYMPTOMS

- mild (6 – 24 hours after last drink)
  - sinus tachycardia
  - systolic hypertension
  - agitation and restlessness
  - tremor
  - insomnia
  - hyperactive reflexes
  - diaphoresis
  - headache
  - nausea and vomiting
- severe
  - hallucinations (12 – 48 hours after last drink)
  - tonic-clonic seizures (6 – 48 hours after last drink)
- delirium tremens (DTs) (72 – 96 hours after last drink)
  - anxiety
  - tachycardia
  - hypertension
  - ataxia
  - diaphoresis

ASSESSMENT

The CLINICAL INSTITUTE WITHDRAWAL ASSESSMENT (CIWA) is a ten-item scale used to objectively assess withdrawal symptoms and ensure withdrawing patients are given the correct amount of medication. Patients are given a score of 0 to 7 for each symptom, based on its severity, except orientation, which is scored from 0 to 4.

- nausea and emesis
- paroxysmal sweats
- level of anxiety
- level of agitation
- tremors
- headache symptoms
- auditory disturbances
- visual disturbances
- tactile disturbances
- orientation

The numerical values for the sections are totaled and the number is used to guide the use of withdrawal medication.

- < 10: very mild withdrawal
- 10 to 15: mild withdrawal
- 16 to 20: modest withdrawal
- > 20: severe withdrawal

TREATMENT AND MANAGEMENT

- IV fluids and electrolytes as needed
- treat for vitamin deficiencies and malnutrition with glucose, thiamine, folate, parenteral multivitamins
- benzodiazepines for agitation
- lorazepam for seizures
- for severe drug-resistant DTs: drug "cocktail" that includes lorazepam, diazepam, and midazolam (Versed) or propofol

QUICK REVIEW QUESTION

6. A 45-year-old man is admitted to the ED with vomiting, profuse sweating, and complaint of a headache. Assessment shows a HR of 130 bpm and blood pressure of 130/102 mm Hg. The nurse checks the patient's chart and notes that the patient has a history of alcohol abuse. What should the nurse prepare to do next?

Opioid Withdrawal

PATHOPHYSIOLOGY

OPIOIDS are synthetically and naturally occurring substances that bind to opioid receptors in the brain, depressing the central nervous system. (The term "opiate" is sometimes used to refer only to naturally occurring opioids.) Chronic use of opioids increases excitability of noradrenergic neurons, and withdrawal leads to hypersensitivity of the central nervous system. Opioid withdrawal is rarely fatal, but death can occur, usually as a result of hemodynamic instability or electrolyte imbalances.

HELPFUL HINT
Commonly used opioids include codeine, fentanyl, heroin, hydrocodone, hydromorphone, meperidine, methadone, morphine, and oxycodone.

ASSESSMENT

The **CLINICAL OPIATE WITHDRAWAL SCALE (COWS)** is an 11-item scale to help objectively assess withdrawal symptoms and ensure that patients are given the correct amount of medication.

Patients are given a score based on the severity of each symptom.

- resting heart rate
- sweating
- restlessness
- pupil size
- bone or joint aches
- rhinorrhea or lacrimation
- GI upset
- tremor
- yawning
- anxiety or irritability
- piloerection

The numerical values for the sections are totaled and the amount is used to guide the use of withdrawal medication.

- 5 – 12: mild withdrawal
- 13 – 24: moderate withdrawal
- 25 – 36: moderate to severe withdrawal
- 36: severe withdrawal

TREATMENT AND MANAGEMENT

- supportive care for symptoms
  - □ benzodiazepines for anxiety, tachycardia, and hypertension
  - □ antiemetics
  - □ clonidine for tachycardia and hypertension
  - □ antidiarrheals
- opioid antagonists: naltrexone and naloxone block the effects of opioids
- opioid replacement therapy: methadone or buprenorphine relieve symptoms without producing intoxication

QUICK REVIEW QUESTION

7. The nurse takes the vitals of a patient in the ED who was admitted for opioid withdrawal. The patient's HR is 102 bpm and her blood pressure is 110/105 mm Hg. What should the nurse anticipate will be ordered for this patient?

ANSWER KEY

1. Inducing vomiting is contraindicated when a patient ingests a caustic agent. Causing regurgitation will re-expose the upper GI tract to the caustic agent.

2. Unlike smoke from fire, which is lighter than air and rises, carbon monoxide mixes with air. Due to this property, the best placement for a carbon monoxide meter is 5 feet off the ground. By the time there is enough carbon monoxide in a room to trigger an alarm placed on the ceiling, there are lethal levels of carbon monoxide in the room.

3. Nurses should consider cyanide toxicity when patients present to the ED after being around a fire: inhaled fumes from burning polymer products such as vinyl and polyurethane will produce cyanide poisoning. Cyanide toxicity can also be caused by a nitroprusside IV infusion.

4. The patient's s/s and history suggest anticholinergic overdose. The nurse should expect to administer physostigmine as an antidote.

5. Opioid overdose can quickly lead to respiratory distress. Administer oxygen and intubate and provide mechanical ventilation if needed.

6. The nurse should anticipate assessing the patient using the CIWA scale and administering medications per the ED's protocol.

7. The nurse should anticipate administering clonidine to the patient for hypertension and tachycardia.

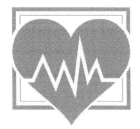

16

COMMUNICABLE DISEASES

BCEN CONTENT OUTLINE

A. *C. Difficile*

★ **B. CHILDHOOD DISEASES** (e.g., measles, mumps, pertussis, chicken pox, diphtheria)

C. Herpes zoster

D. Mononucleosis

★ **E. MULTI-DRUG RESISTANT ORGANISMS** (e.g., MRSA, VRE)

F. Tuberculosis

ISOLATION PRECAUTIONS

PURPOSE

ISOLATION PRECAUTIONS are used to prevent the spread of infection. The precautions are guidelines set by organizations like the World Health Organization (WHO) and the Centers for Disease Control (CDC) to prevent the transmission of microorganisms that are responsible for causing infection. There are two tiers of isolation precautions: the first tier is standard precautions, and the second tier consists of three transmission precautions (airborne, droplet, and contact).

STANDARD PRECAUTIONS

- Assume that all patients are carrying a microorganism.
- Practice hand hygiene.
- Wear gloves.
- Prevent needle sticks.
- Avoid splash and spray; wear appropriate PPE if there is a possibility of body fluids splashing or spraying.

AIRBORNE PRECAUTIONS

- Patient should be placed in a private room with a negative-pressure air system and the door kept closed.

- Wear N95 respirator mask; place on before entering the room and keep on until after leaving the room.

- Place N95 or surgical mask on patient during transport.

DROPLET PRECAUTIONS

- Place patient in a private room; the door may remain open.

- Wear appropriate PPE within 3 feet of patient.

- Wash hands with antimicrobial soap after removing gloves and mask, before leaving the patient's room.

- Place surgical mask on patient during transport.

CONTACT PRECAUTIONS

- Place the patient in a private room; the door may remain open.

- Change gloves after touching infected materials.

- Remove gloves before leaving patient's room.

- Wear gown; remove before leaving patient's room.

- Use patient-dedicated equipment if possible; community equipment is to be used clean and disinfected between patients.

- During transport keep precautions in place and notify different areas as needed.

QUICK REVIEW QUESTION

1. The nurse is assigned to a patient who has a positive diagnosis of measles. What PPE should the nurse wear?

C. DIFFICILE

PATHOPHYSIOLOGY

DID YOU KNOW?
Proton inhibitors and H2 blockers have both been shown to be risk factors for C. diff infection.

Clostridium difficile (commonly called ***C. diff***) is an acute bacterial infection in the intestine most commonly seen after antibiotic use. The antibiotics disrupt the normal intestinal flora, allowing the antibiotic-resistant C. diff spores to proliferate in the intestines. The bacterium releases a toxin that causes the intestine to produce yellow-white plaques on the intestinal lining. The C. diff infection can produce inflammation in the intestines, resulting in toxic colitis (toxic megacolon) or pseudomembranous colitis, and may also lead to perforation and sepsis.

TRANSMISSION AND PRECAUTIONS

- fecal to oral transmission
- use contact precautions
- do not use foams and gels (they will not kill the spores)
- environmental cleanse of a 1:10 bleach-to-water solution

DIAGNOSIS

- foul-smelling diarrhea 5 – 10 days after start of antibiotic
- s/s of toxic colitis: tenesmus, rectal bleeding, abdominal distension and tenderness
- enzyme immunoassay (EIA): most commonly run diagnostic test
- PCR test on the stool specimen: most sensitive and specific diagnostic test

TREATMENT AND MANAGEMENT

- antibiotic-induced *C. diff*: stop current use of antibiotics if possible
- oral antibiotics; IV if oral antibiotics cannot be tolerated
  - □ vancomycin (Vancocin)
  - □ fidaxomicin (Dificid)
  - □ metronidazole (Flagyl)

QUICK REVIEW QUESTION

2. A patient is admitted to the ED with a suspected *C. difficile* infection. What PPE should the nurse use?

CHILDHOOD DISEASES ★

- **CHICKEN POX** (varicella zoster virus) is a viral infection that infects the conjunctiva or the mucous membranes of the upper respiratory tract. The infection then spreads, causing the hallmark rash of small, itchy, fluid-filled blisters all over the body.
  - □ Transmissions and Precautions: person-to-person through direct contact or airborne droplets; airborne, droplet, and contact precautions
  - □ Diagnosis: itchy rash that forms small fluid-filled blisters that eventually scab; mild headache; moderate fever; fatigue; varicella titer test on a blood sample; Tzanck test performed on a swab sample of the lesion area
  - □ Management: supportive care for symptoms (systemic antihistamines, colloidal oatmeal baths); antivirals in severe cases

- **DIPHTHERIA** is an infection caused by the bacterium *Corynebacterium diphtheriae*. The bacterium enters through the pharynx or the skin and releases a toxin that causes inflammation and necrosis.
  - □ Transmissions and Precautions: person-to-person through respiratory droplets (pharyngeal infection); person-to-person skin contact (skin infection); droplet, contact precautions
  - □ Diagnosis: white or gray glossy exudate in the back of the throat; mild sore throat; serosanguinous or purulent discharge; difficulty swallowing or getting food stuck in throat; hoarseness; edema, visibly swollen neck (bull neck); stridor; low-grade fever; skin infection presents with non-specific symptoms; positive culture from swab
  - □ Management: diphtheria antitoxin (IM or IV); antibiotics (penicillin, erythromycin); clean skin infection with soap and water; diphtheria vaccination after recovery

- **MEASLES** is an acute infection caused by a paramyxovirus. The virus enters through the upper respiratory tract or conjunctiva and spreads systemically through the lymph nodes, triggering a systemic inflammatory response.
  - □ Transmissions and Precautions: person to person through respiratory droplets that can live in the air or on hard surfaces for up to 2 hours; airborne, droplet, and contact precautions
  - □ Diagnosis: fever; cough; runny nose; conjunctivitis; sore throat; Koplik spots; cephalocaudal rash (usually starts behind the ears); positive PCR or serum measles IgM antibody
  - □ Management: vitamin A; supportive care for symptoms

- **MUMPS** is an acute infection caused by a paramyxovirus. The virus is an inflammatory response that results in swelling of the salivary glands (usually the parotid glands).
  - □ Transmissions and Precautions: person to person through respiratory droplets in close proximity; droplet precautions
  - □ Diagnosis: fever; salivary gland edema; parotitis; pain when chewing or swallowing; swelling in submandibular glands or tongue; positive serum IgM or PCR
  - □ Management: supportive care for symptoms; isolate until glandular swelling is gone

- **PERTUSSIS** (whooping cough) is an infection caused by the bacterium *Bordetella pertussis* that causes a mucopurulent sanguineous exudate that can compromise the respiratory tract.
  - □ Transmissions and Precautions: person to person through respiratory droplets in close proximity; droplet precautions
  - □ Diagnosis: paroxysmal or spasmodic cough ("whoop") that ends in a prolonged, high-pitched inspiration; PCR on nasal or throat swab
  - □ Management: antibiotics (erythromycin, azithromycin); supportive care for symptoms, including suctioning

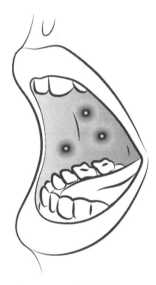

Figure 16.1. Koplik Spots

DID YOU KNOW?

Children with viral infections should not be given aspirin: it increases these children's risk of developing **Reye's syndrome**, a life-threatening encephalopathy linked to viral infections and aspirin use.

3. A mother brings her 2-year-old into the ED with complaints of a persistent cough and hoarseness. What tests should the nurse anticipate to determine if the child has pertussis?

HERPES ZOSTER

PATHOPHYSIOLOGY

HERPES ZOSTER, more commonly known as SHINGLES, is an acute viral infection that is the result of the varicella zoster virus reactivating in a posterior dorsal root ganglion. The varicella zoster virus initially infects most patients as children during an episode of chicken pox. In adulthood, the virus comes out of latency and inflames the sensory root ganglion, the dermatome, and the skin associated with the dermatome.

TRANSMISSION AND PRECAUTIONS

- contact with fluid from blisters caused by rash
- before blisters appear and after blisters are completely dry and crusted: standard precautions
- before blisters are completely dry and crusted: airborne and contact precautions

DIAGNOSIS

- redness and rash of blisters: linear on one side of the body, usually in the truncal area
- sharp, burning pain with tingling or itching
- Tzanck test can be performed on a swab sample of the lesion area

TREATMENT AND MANAGEMENT

- oral or IV antivirals (acyclovir [Zovirax], famciclovir [Famvir], valacyclovir [Valtrex])
- wet compress on blister area
- pain management
  - □ systemically with gabapentin (Neurontin) or cyclic antidepressants
  - □ locally with topical capsaicin or xylocaine (Lidocaine) ointment

QUICK REVIEW QUESTION

4. A topical analgesic has been applied to a patient with shingles, but the patient still complains of pain. What medication should the nurse expect to administer to the patient?

MONONUCLEOSIS

PATHOPHYSIOLOGY

MONONUCLEOSIS, commonly known as mono, is an infection caused by the Epstein-Barr virus. The virus replicates in the epithelial cells of the pharynx and in B lymphocytes, triggering a response from the body's immune system. Mono is common in children and presents with mild symptoms. Symptoms can be more severe in young and older adults.

TRANSMISSION AND PRECAUTIONS

- most commonly transmitted through saliva
- contact precautions

DIAGNOSIS

- fatigue lasting from a few weeks to months
- fever
- pharyngitis
- palatal petechiae
- lymphadenopathy
- adenopathy
- splenic rupture
- mononuclear spot test (usually Monospot)

HELPFUL HINT
Due to risk of splenic rupture, avoid deep pressure palpation of the abdomen in patients with mononucleosis.

TREATMENT AND MANAGEMENT

- supportive treatment for symptoms
- discharge teaching: rest, avoid heavy lifting and contact sports for 1 month or until splenomegaly resolves

QUICK REVIEW QUESTION

5. A patient arrives at the ED with symptoms of mononucleosis. What should the nurse avoid while assessing the patient?

★ MULTI-DRUG-RESISTANT ORGANISMS

- **METHICILLIN-RESISTANT *Staphylococcus aureus* (MRSA)** is a bacterial infection caused by a strain of *Staphylococcus* ("staph") that is resistant to many of the antibiotics normally used to treat staph infections, including the beta-lactam agents ampicillin, amoxicillin, methicillin, penicillin, and cephalosporin.
  - ☐ Diagnosis: red area on the skin; swelling; pain; warm to the touch; pus or drainage from bumps on skin; fever; positive culture of MRSA bacterium

- Management: antibiotics (trimethoprim, sulfamethoxazole, clindamycin linezolid)
- **VANCOMYCIN-RESISTANT ENTEROCOCCI (VRE)** is a bacterial infection caused by strains of enterococci bacteria that are resistant to vancomycin.
  - Diagnosis: s/s of wound infection, pneumonia, UTI, meningitis, or sepsis; culture and sensitivity
  - Management (general): antibiotics (amoxicillin, ampicillin, gentamicin, penicillin, piperacillin, streptomycin)
  - Management (skin infections): daptomycin, linezolid, tedizolid, tigecycline
  - Management (intra-abdominal infections): piperacillin-tazobactam, imipenem, meropenem

QUICK REVIEW QUESTION

6. Which antibiotics should NOT be used to treat patients with methicillin-resistant *Staphylococcus aureus* (MRSA)?

TUBERCULOSIS

PATHOPHYSIOLOGY

TUBERCULOSIS (TB) is a chronic, progressive bacterial infection of the lungs. There is an initial asymptomatic infection followed by a period of latency that may develop into active disease. Active TB produces granulomatous necrosis, more commonly known as lesions. The rupturing of the lesions in the pleural space can cause empyema, bronchopleural fistulas, or a pneumothorax.

TRANSMISSION AND PRECAUTIONS

- person-to-person through respiratory droplets
- airborne precautions
- prolonged productive cough
- fever and fatigue
- night sweats
- hemoptysis
- dyspnea
- TB skin test (Mantoux skin test)
- chest X-ray showing multinodular infiltrate near the clavicle

TREATMENT AND MANAGEMENT

- supportive treatment for symptoms
- 2 months of treatment with: isoniazid (INH), rifampin (RIF), pyrazinamide (PZA), ethambutol (EMB)

- After 2 months of treatment, PZA and EMB discontinued after 2 months; INH and RIF continue for another 4 – 7 months

QUICK REVIEW QUESTION

7. A patient in the ED complains of a cough that has lasted for several weeks and also states that they have been waking up at night covered in sweat. Which diagnostic test should the nurse prepare for?

ANSWER KEY

1. The nurse should use gloves and an N95 respirator.

2. *C. difficile* requires contact protections, so the nurse should use gloves and an isolation gown.

3. The diagnostic tests for pertussis include nasopharyngeal culture and PCR testing. The PCR test is preferred because it is the most sensitive.

4. The nurse should expect to administer gabapentin, which treats neuropathic pain.

5. The nurse should avoid deep abdominal palpation due to the risk of splenic rupture in patients with mononucleosis.

6. MRSA is resistant to beta-lactam agents, including ampicillin, amoxicillin, methicillin, penicillin, and cephalosporin.

7. The nurse should prepare the patient for a chest X-ray to confirm tuberculosis.

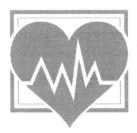

17

PROFESSIONAL ISSUES

BCEN CONTENT OUTLINE

A. Nurse
1. Critical Incident Stress Management
★ **2. ETHICAL DILEMMAS**
3. Evidence-based practice
4. Lifelong learning
5. Research

B. Patient
1. Discharge planning
★ **2. END OF LIFE ISSUES**
3. Forensic evidence collection
4. Pain management and procedural sedation
5. Patient safety
6. Patient satisfaction
7. Transfer and stabilization
★ **8. TRANSITIONS OF CARE**
★ **9. CULTURAL CONSIDERATIONS** (e.g., interpretive services, privacy, decision-making)

C. System
1. Delegation of tasks to assistive personnel
2. Disaster management (i.e., preparedness, mitigation, response, and recovery)
3. Federal regulations (e.g., HIPAA, EMTALA)
4. Patient consent for treatment
5. Performance improvement
★ **6. RISK MANAGEMENT**
7. Symptom surveillance

D. Triage

NURSE

Critical Incident Stress Management

CRITICAL INCIDENTS are sudden and unexpected events that can impact an individual or group in such a way that it overwhelms the ability of the individual or group to cope, resulting in significant psychological distress. CRITICAL INCIDENT STRESS MANAGEMENT (CISM) programs are comprehensive, with the goal of helping personnel return to a baseline state of emotional health. There are several components to a CISM system:

- precrisis preparation
- demobilization and consultation
- defusing
- critical incident stress debriefing
- crisis intervention
- family CISM
- follow-up

Debriefing is a key element to CISM, and can occur immediately after the event, or as soon as it is possible to assemble all key players (up to 14 days later).

- provides perspective and closure for staff involved
- prevents personal feelings of blame or responsibility
- opens discussion for improvement for future events

QUICK REVIEW QUESTION

1. A charge nurse in the ED notices that a new nurse in the department is withdrawn, quiet, and struggling to keep up with tasks in her assignment. The charge knows this nurse experienced her first pediatric resuscitation on the previous shift, and there was a poor outcome. What can the charge do to help this nurse?

★ Ethical Dilemmas

ETHICAL DILEMMAS are situations that require healthcare providers to balance competing ethical principles; such situations are present in all areas of healthcare. Ethical dilemmas that occur in the emergency department include decisional capacity determination, medical futility considerations, and refusals of care.

DECISIONAL CAPACITY relates to the expectation that patients have a responsibility to participate in their own care, whenever able. Decisional capacity is fluid and can change based on the patient's presentation and status throughout emergency care. If decisional capacity is determined to be diminished, a surrogate or medical power of attorney may be used. DIMINISHED DECISIONAL CAPACITY can be due to several factors:

- alcohol intoxication
- trauma
- sedation

DID YOU KNOW?
Diminished decisional capacity can be reversed. For example, a patient with hypoxia may regain decisional capacity after the underlying medical condition is corrected.

- extreme stress
- hypoxia
- developmental delay

Assessment of decisional capacity is based on the patient's:

- ability to provide an accurate and detailed medical history
- cooperation with the physical evaluation
- understanding of the recommended treatments

In cases of acute emergency, when there is no time to obtain consent from the patient, implied consent is understood. **IMPLIED CONSENT** is the assumption that a rational human being wants to live as long as possible.

MEDICAL FUTILITY refers to medical interventions in emergency situations that are not likely to result in significant positive outcomes for the patient. Interventions that are futile are characterized as ones that maintain permanent states of unconsciousness.

In the ED setting, there are some interventions that are carried out automatically, even in the absence of a medical history.

- CPR
- fluid resuscitation (blood products in the presence of hemorrhagic shock)
- intubation and ventilation in respiratory distress or arrest

If a case of futility is questioned, the ED healthcare team should act in line with the standard ethical principles for medical and nursing practice. If there is time, an ethics committee can be convened to assist with decision-making in cases such as these.

Patients who have intact decisional capacity have the **RIGHT TO REFUSE ANY AND ALL CARE**. The responsibility of the ED nurse is to provide the patient with as much information as they can to allow the patient to make an informed decision to refuse care. This applies to surrogates or family members responsible for making care decisions as well.

LEAVING AGAINST MEDICAL ADVICE (AMA) is when a patient requests to leave the care of the emergency physician and depart the ED. If the patient chooses to do so, the physician will counsel the patient on the risks of such a departure, and then ask the patient to provide a signature acknowledging these risks.

INVOLUNTARY COMMITMENT is a legal process under which a physician determines that a patient is unsafe to themselves or others and requires close observation under medical care for the sake of safety. State laws govern involuntary commitment and should be reviewed prior to involuntarily committing a patient to care.

Decisions in these cases are made based on the ethical principles of autonomy, beneficence, non-maleficence, justice, and veracity.

- **AUTONOMY**: Recognition that a patient is a unique individual with the right to have their own opinions, values, beliefs, and perspectives. Nurses advocate for patients without judgment, coercion, or assertion of the nurse's own beliefs or values.

- **BENEFICENCE:** Acting with the intent of doing good or the right thing. This principle addresses the obligation to act in the best interest of the patient when there may be other competing interests.

- **NON-MALEFICENCE:** "Do no harm." This principle relates to the nurse's responsibility to protect the public and the patient from harm in the context of the care setting.

- **JUSTICE:** Provision of equitable access to care. This principle covers providing care to all patients regardless of socioeconomic status, insurance coverage, or any other demographic category.

- **VERACITY:** The practice of complete truthfulness with patients and families.

QUICK REVIEW QUESTION

2. An adult patient arrives at the ED with evidence of polytrauma, and CPR is in progress. The emergency physician and trauma surgeon disagree on the futility of further intervention. How can the charge nurse help address the situation?

Evidence-Based Practice

EVIDENCE-BASED PRACTICE **(EBP)** is the use of high-quality research outcomes to inform clinical practice. EBP is typically implemented through the establishment of a CLINICAL PRACTICE GUIDELINE **(CPG)**, either at the local organization or professional association (such as the Emergency Nurses Association) level. EBP is developed based on a combination of research data and evidence and clinical experience meeting the needs of a specific organization.

Nurses have a responsibility to practice with the most up-to-date evidence guiding them. However, implementation of such practice is not done on an individual basis and should be a collaborative effort within the disciplines of healthcare.

There are many types of research. The following types are listed in order of the value of the evidence that comes from them. The first listed are generally recognized as providing the highest level of evidence and are therefore the most useful in the EBP implementation process.

- Systematic reviews and meta-analysis (quantitative) are the most reliable sources of evidence, and practice policies or guidelines can be based on them.

- Randomized controlled trials (quantitative) are used in medical research more often than in nursing research, but they are the standard method when studying very specific interventions, such as in pharmacological research.

- Cohort studies (quantitative) compare two groups of subjects, one with and one without a certain characteristic, over time. Comparisons are made in order to predict the outcomes based on demographic and other variables.

- Qualitative studies collect the thoughts, feelings, and perspectives of patients concerning a topic; the results are then used to inform practice.

■ Case studies are presentations of interesting patient cases, typically written by providers.

There are steps to implementing research into EBP. Two models used for such implementation are the Iowa and Stetler models.

■ The IOWA MODEL is a seven-step process: identifying a problem, forming a team, collecting evidence, grading the evidence, creating a CPG, implementing it, and evaluating it.

■ The STETLER MODEL is a five-step process: preparation, validation, comparative evaluation, translation, and evaluation.

QUICK REVIEW QUESTION

3. An ED nurse is noted to have tried new nursing interventions that are not in the current local CPG. When approached, the nurse says, "I read an article that said this improves patient outcomes." Why were these actions inappropriate?

Research

Emergency nurses who choose to read research studies to inform their personal practice must know how to identify reliable sources of evidence. An assessment should be done on each article read to determine if it is valid and reliable. Consider the following questions:

■ Is the evidence recent, published within the last 5 – 7 years?

■ Was it carried out in an ethical, legal manner?

■ Was the design appropriate for the research question?

■ Was the population chosen appropriate to the research question?

■ Was the sample size adequate?

■ Was a literature review performed?

■ If instruments were used, were they validated?

■ Do the findings address the current clinical problem?

Nursing research conducted in EDs must follow all ethical and legal regulations in order to be done reliably and correctly. Emergency nurses interested in performing research typically follow a continuum of nursing research.

■ understand research concepts

■ critique research for use in practice

■ systematically review the literature on a topic

■ participate in clinical-practice change projects

■ participate in a research study

■ act as primary investigator in a nursing research study

QUICK REVIEW QUESTION

4. How can emergency nurses demonstrate interest in the research process and join a research protocol in the agency?

Lifelong Learning

Emergency nursing is a specialty practice that must be promoted within the overall profession of nursing. Professional nursing associations advance their mission and vision statements and establish standards of professional practice.

CERTIFICATION in the specialty demonstrates a commitment to the profession and to lifelong learning and growth within the discipline. Earning **CONTINUING EDUCATION** credits demonstrates current practice knowledge and is often required for licensure and recertification in the specialty. Examples of continuing education activity include:

- conference attendance
- webinar participation
- lunch-and-learn participation
- grand rounds presentations
- higher-level nursing education (BSN, MSN, DNP, PhD)

QUICK REVIEW QUESTION

5. How can an emergency nurse demonstrate continuing education to licensing bodies and to prospective employers?

PATIENT

Discharge Planning and Transitions of Care

DID YOU KNOW?
Emergency nurses can offer community resources to patients who are homeless or otherwise require assistance, but this should not prevent discharge from the ED of an otherwise healthy patient.

DISCHARGE PLANNING in the setting of the ED generally consists of arranging for follow-up care either with primary care services or specialty care consultations. Patients discharged from the ED are considered stable and should not require extensive discharge planning services. Effective **CARE COORDINATION**—the organization of patient care activities between two medical entities (ED and primary care, community care, etc.)—can help prevent over-reliance on ED and urgent care settings.

TRANSITION OF CARE is the process of moving patients from one care setting to another. Key considerations for transitions of care include:

- accessibility of services
- information sharing and communication
- community partnerships
- care coordination
- health care utilization and costs
- safety

QUICK REVIEW QUESTION

6. What is the role of the emergency nurse in the transition of care for patients seen in the ED?

Organic and Tissue Donation

ORGAN AND TISSUE DONATION is an important step in end-of-life care in the ED. When a patient dies, there is only a short window of time in which to arrange for donation; certain steps are required to do so successfully.

The steps to successful procurement are as follows:

- **DETERMINATION OF DEATH**, followed by **DECLARATION OF DEATH**. Brain death is generally declared if there are fixed pupils, an absence of reflexes in the brain stem, or no respiratory effort, or if tests have confirmed the absence of perfusion or electrical activity in the brain tissue.

- **MEDICAL EXAMINER REVIEW AND APPROVAL**. Depending on the mechanism of the patient's death, the medical examiner may need to grant approval for organ procurement. (This requirement is governed by state laws and may vary.) Examples of such situations include suicide, homicide, accidental death, pediatric death, and death after admission to hospital or long-term care facility.

- **NOTIFICATION OF LOCAL ORGAN PROCUREMENT ORGANIZATION**. The procurement organization should be called in every event.

- **REVIEW OF PATIENT CONSENT OR WISHES**. There are circumstances in which the patient's wishes are clear, such as in advance directives, a will, or indication on the driver's license. In these cases, no further consent is needed. If the patient's preference is unclear, the legal next of kin must provide consent.

The process of organ procurement can be a long one due to these steps and other factors. Care of the patient awaiting procurement must consider the preservation of tissues. The following parameters are preferred (in the case of patients in a vegetative state but still functionally alive).

- Maintain intravascular volume when possible.

- Maintain vital signs within normal limits to include temperature.

- Promote diuresis if possible.

- Manage tissue oxygenation and acid-base balance.

If the patient is not in a vegetative state, but tissue is still eligible for donation (eye donors) follow these parameters:

- Maintain the head of the bed at 20 degrees.

- Instill artificial tears or saline to preserve tissue.

- Tape eyes closed using paper tape, and place compresses over eyes to deter swelling.

QUICK REVIEW QUESTION

7. A patient has been declared brain dead in the ED, but is still hemodynamically stable via mechanical ventilation. What steps should the nurse take following the declaration of brain death?

HELPFUL HINT

Typically, the organ and tissue procurement agency is called for every death in the ED to determine if the patient is eligible for procurement. The agency will usually speak with family members to discuss donation.

Advance Directives

ADVANCE DIRECTIVES are written statements of individuals' wishes with regard to medical treatment decisions such as resuscitation, intubation, and other interventions. They are made to ensure the wishes of the individual are carried out in the event the person is unable to express those wishes at the time of care.

Advance directives must be valid, up to date, and documented before they can be honored in the ED. In order to honor an advance directive, the physician must see the paperwork, validate the paperwork, and place an order that indicates the advance directive status of the patient.

Advance directives generally dictate the level of life-saving measures taken in certain circumstances.

- **DO NOT RESUSCITATE (DNR)** typically indicates that no heroic measures should be taken to sustain the patient's life.

- **DO NOT INTUBATE (DNI)** indicates that the patient does not wish to be intubated if the need presents.

- **ALLOW NATURAL DEATH (AND)** indicates the patient does not want any intervention that may sustain life or prevent a natural progression to death.

Any combination of DNR, DNI, and AND may be requested, and other requests may be present in the documentation if applicable to the patient's circumstance.

LIVING WILLS are also used in situations where a patient may have a terminal illness or is acutely in a vegetative state. They allow an individual to state which treatments they would like in the event they are unable to express such at the time of illness.

DURABLE POWERS OF ATTORNEY or **MEDICAL POWERS OF ATTORNEY** may also be used in situations at the end of life. A power of attorney designates an individual to make decisions in place of the patient when the patient does not have the capacity to do so. It may be general or very specific in the range of decisions this surrogate can make.

Decisions to withhold, withdraw, or transition to palliative care are typically made before or after an ED visit. If circumstances present that necessitate such decisions, conformity to living wills, advance directives, and powers of attorney must occur. In the absence of legal documentation to guide such decisions, a multidisciplinary approach should be taken to inform patients and families of options for these decisions.

QUICK REVIEW QUESTION

8. An 85-year-old patient arrives at the ED for nausea and dizziness. Soon after arrival, the patient becomes unresponsive and requires CPR. Her daughter states the patient does not wish to be resuscitated. What should the ED nurse do next?

Family Presence

Family presence in the ED, particularly during procedures or resuscitation, is a complex and controversial topic. Generally, family presence, even during invasive procedure and resuscitation, is recommended. Evidence shows that family members assert that it is their preference and right to be present for these efforts, especially in the case of pediatric care.

Family member presence should be offered if appropriate and should be governed by local policy and guidelines for consistency and provision of boundaries. However, if a family member is behaving inappropriately or interfering with care, they should not be present.

HELPFUL HINT
Family members may find their experience in the ED difficult, and a staff member should be assigned to be available to discuss the events occurring. A chaplain or other community support staff may also be requested.

QUICK REVIEW QUESTION

9. An emergency nurse is assigned to assist a family as they witness the resuscitation of their loved one. The outcome is poor, and the patient does not survive. The family asks what happens to the patient next. What should the nurse tell the family?

Forensic Evidence Collection

FORENSIC EVIDENCE COLLECTION occurs in the emergency setting when a crime is known or suspected to have been committed, and collection of evidence is vital to the care of the patient and potential victims. Situations in which forensic evidence may be collected include:

- GSWs
- trauma
- sexual assault
- domestic abuse
- child abuse

Evidence collection should be systematic and done with high accountability for detail and inventory. The ED nurse must have a solid understanding of collection techniques and chain-of-custody considerations. While processes vary with local regulations, some general guidelines are given below.

- Place clean sheets or other clean barrier on the floor or a large table. (Barrier will be submitted as evidence.)
- Remove clothing one article at a time by cutting, being careful to avoid any tears, bullet holes, or obviously soiled areas to prevent deterioration of evidence on the clothing.
- Paper bags must be used for packaging. Package each item or article separately. Avoid excessive handling of evidence.
- Retrieve non-clothing evidence and seal in appropriate bag or envelope.
- Collect evidence from gunshot wounds.
- Cover victim's hands, if possible, to preserve gunpowder residue if it is present.

- If the bullet is retained, or found in the clothing, handle it as little as possible and seal in the appropriate container.

- Collect evidence from under fingernails by scraping the contents under the nail onto a white sheet of paper to be folded and placed in an envelope as described above.

- Evidence of suspected or reported bodily fluids should be removed with a cotton-tipped applicator. Allow the swab tip to dry, and place in a signed, sealed envelope.

- Document chain of custody.

Label the evidence (every item) using the appropriate form. When the evidence is given to law enforcement, an inventory of the items and the officer's ID should be documented in the medical record.

SEXUAL ASSAULT NURSE EXAMINERS (SANE NURSES) are registered nurses who have completed specialized certification and training for clinical practice in medical forensic care of victims and alleged perpetrators. They should be used whenever possible to collect evidence for a rape kit. It is best practice to use this resource due to the sensitivity and obligation to collect the evidence in a careful manner.

QUICK REVIEW QUESTION

10. The nurse is supervising a technician as he cuts away clothing on a trauma patient. She notes that the technician is cutting the clothing with no regard for evidence that may be retained on the garments. How should the nurse approach this issue?

Pain Management and Procedural Sedation

PAIN MANAGEMENT in the ED is a complex and controversial issue in the context of the current opioid crisis facing the United States. Both non-pharmacological and pharmacological approaches to pain should be considered.

- Non-pharmacological interventions include repositioning the patient; keeping the patient relaxed or distracted; and applying ice, heat, or massage.

- Pharmacological interventions include acetaminophen, NSAIDs, opioids, muscle relaxants, and local anesthetics.

Nurses are charged with managing expectations for pain relief with patients. Nursing considerations for the care of patients in pain:

- Pain assessment is a numerical score as well as a subjective description of the nature of pain from a patient's perspective.

- Measurement of pain should occur as frequently as every measurement of vital signs, or more frequently if indicated.

- Patients may have unrealistic expectations of pain management and will need education on the subject. Establishing a goal for pain with the patient may help mitigate this issue.

PROCEDURAL SEDATION in the ED is performed with a sedation-certified registered nurse, the emergency physician, and occasionally a consult such as cardiology,

DID YOU KNOW?
It's a common myth that some patients feel less pain; however, medication should never be withheld from a patient based on the patient's race, age, religion, gender identity, or cognitive ability.

orthopedics, or general surgery. It is indicated for anxiolysis, analgesia, and amnesia for uncomfortable procedures that do not require general anesthesia or admission to the operating room (e.g., synchronized cardioversion, reduction of fractures).

The ED nurse's role in procedural sedation is to assist during the procedure and help the patient recover. Nurses should confirm that all consents are in place before beginning and participate in the time-out and debriefing before and after the procedure.

QUICK REVIEW QUESTION

11. A pediatric patient's mother asks about the procedural sedation process for her son who was climbing a fence, fell, and broke his arm. She is concerned that the procedure should be performed in the operating room, and does not feel comfortable with it happening in the ED. How can the nurse respond to this mother?

Patient Safety and Risk Management ★

Potential **PATIENT SAFETY** issues in the ED include patient falls, medication errors, and the safety of moderately ill patients in waiting rooms.

- **PREVENTING FALLS** in the ED is a difficult endeavor due to the chaotic and fast-paced nature of the work. Communication with the patient, provision of call lights, and hourly rounding are good ways to mitigate the risk of patient falls.

- **MEDICATION ERRORS** in emergency situations or resuscitation efforts are at a greater risk of occurring in the ED. Drills and practice in these situations allow the nurse to be confident and efficient in administering emergency drugs.

- ED **OVERCROWDING** can lead to poor patient outcomes in the waiting room before a patient can be seen. Hourly rounding and reassessment of patients can prevent deterioration or waiting room deaths.

RISK MANAGERS typically assess risk in the hospital system or agency overall. However, they will also assess certain events occurring in the ED: adverse or sentinel events, or any patient complaint or concern that might lead to litigation. Risk managers then perform formal root-cause analysis of these cases to identify what led to the poor outcome. **ROOT-CAUSE ANALYSIS** is a stepwise process.

- examines policy compliance or presence of standard operating procedures to govern processes

- considers decision-making leading up to the event

- establishes a sequence of events or a timeline leading to the event

- considers individuals or groups of individuals involved

- often done in focus group setting with multidisciplinary participation

- may take several months to complete the investigation

12. An ED nurse identifies a near-miss event that could have resulted in a sentinel event for a patient. He asks his nurse manager how to properly report the incident to prevent it from happening again. What is the best response by the nurse manager?

Patient Satisfaction

PATIENT SATISFACTION is measured to determine if and what areas of the overall patient care experience need improvement. Different regulatory bodies may be concerned with patient satisfaction rates, and they use different tools and processes to measure patient satisfaction.

One common patient satisfaction survey is the HOSPITAL CONSUMER ASSESSMENT OF HEALTHCARE PROVIDERS AND SYSTEMS (HCAHPS) survey. The HCAHPS survey addresses over 20 patient perspectives on care and allows the patient to rate their experiences. Scores can be used in the context of quality assurance and performance appraisal and measurement, and as a means to improve on the departmental or unit level.

Patient satisfaction is driven by many variables, some of which are under the control of the department and many of which are not.

- care outcomes
- facility services
- customer service practices
- overall appearance of facility
- attitude/knowledge of staff
- availability of equipment or supplies
- pain management

QUICK REVIEW QUESTION

13. Why are patient satisfaction scores important to nursing in the ED?

Transfer and Stabilization

Transfer and stabilization of patients in the ED is governed by federal regulations in the CONSOLIDATED OMNIBUS BUDGET RECONCILIATION ACT (COBRA), which includes the EMERGENCY MEDICAL TREATMENT AND ACTIVE LABOR ACT (EMTALA). According to EMTALA, any patient presenting to an ED requesting care must at a minimum receive a medical screening exam performed by a qualified medical provider (triage by an RN does not qualify). If the exam reveals a condition requiring immediate or near-immediate care, the following must occur:

- The patient receives care and is discharged to home if stable.
- The patient is admitted to the facility if the appropriate resources are available.

- The patient is transferred to another facility with the appropriate level of care.

Transfers of patients to higher levels of care require the following:

- The patient must be stable for transport.
- There must be an accepting physician at a receiving hospital that has the right services for the care of the patient.
- The risks and benefits of transfer must be disclosed to the patient, and written, informed consent must be signed and sent with the patient.
- Medical records must be sent from the transporting hospital to the destination, and a report must be sent or called in before patient arrives.
- The method of transfer must be appropriate to the scale of the patient's condition.

Transport methods must be appropriate to the patient's needs; excessive cost or use of resources that may be needed elsewhere should be avoided.

- SURFACE TRANSPORT is typically the lowest-cost option; however, it takes the most time. It can accommodate large patients or large equipment and is less affected by weather conditions.
- ROTOR-WING TRANSPORT (helicopters) provides rapid transport from two points, either hospital to hospital or point of injury to hospital. It can be limited by weather conditions and distance between points due to fuel concerns and by weight.
- FIXED-WING TRANSPORT (airplanes) is the most expensive and is used when other modes are not available. It can cover long distances, has a pressurized cabin, and can accommodate gear and people.

Nursing considerations for the care of a patient needing transport include:

- Ensure peripheral or central line access is patent. If peripheral, establish two access sites.
- Decompress gastric gases if patient is transporting via rotor-wing transport.
- Insert urinary catheter.
- Determine if blood products need to be packed and sent with patient or if the crew has their own.
- Consider the impact of higher elevation on equipment and hollow organs. Consider chest tube placement if appropriate for the patient's condition.

QUICK REVIEW QUESTION

14. What is the nurse's role and responsibility in preparing a patient for transfer?

Cultural Considerations ★

CULTURAL CONSIDERATIONS in the context of emergency nursing include respecting cultural practices that inform patients' decisions to accept certain treatments and demonstrating cultural competence in care. Quality care can be achieved when diversity is approached in a nonjudgmental, positive, and sensitive manner.

Areas of diversity to consider include age, race, culture, ethnicity, nationality, gender identity, sexual orientation, religion, and marginalization (those considered by some to be unworthy of care based on actions, like using drugs or having committed a criminal offense). Each area of diversity influences patient and family responses to medical care, medical decision-making, and compliance with care.

QUICK REVIEW QUESTION

15. An emergency nurse encounters a patient with religious beliefs that he is not familiar with. What is the best way to respect the patient's beliefs during the course of care?

SYSTEM

Delegation of Tasks

DELEGATION of tasks is governed by local organizational policies, state nurse practice acts, and professional association practice guidelines. State nurse practice acts outline specific scopes of practice for all licensed personnel working in healthcare settings. Registered nurses in the ED may delegate tasks to the following licensed personnel:

- paramedics and EMTs working in the ED
- LPNs/LVNs
- medical assistants
- nursing assistants
- technicians

Tasks must be delegated with the following understandings:

- Delegation does not take away the nurse's responsibility for the completion of the task and its outcome.
- Delegation should take into account the scope of practice and, to the extent possible, the skills and abilities of the individual to whom the task is delegated.

QUICK REVIEW QUESTION

16. If an ED nurse is unsure what tasks are appropriate to delegate to technicians, where can this information be found?

Disaster Management

DISASTER MANAGEMENT in the context of emergency nursing includes considerations for mass casualty incidents, natural disasters, pandemic/epidemic illness, and decontamination of patients. DISASTER PREPAREDNESS is usually managed in the form of large-scale drills or tabletop exercises to determine how to mitigate weaknesses and identify needs in disaster management plans.

Many organizations use the INCIDENT COMMAND SYSTEM (ICS) promoted by FEMA to manage disaster situations. Each role in the ICS is preassigned and drilled in preparation for disaster events. Organizations may customize the hierarchy below the general staff to fit the needs of their own system.

The following are four steps to disaster management and preparedness.

- Mitigation: Identify vulnerabilities to threats or weaknesses in current plans.

- Preparedness: Develop mutual aid agreements, create disaster management plans, determine supply thresholds and needs, consider stockpiles, and establish a command and control structure.

- Response: Warn (notify), isolate (during the disaster), and rescue (following the disaster).

- Recovery: Inventory supplies and resources, relieve staff members present during the isolation phase, incorporate records into the EMR, implement CISM program if needed, and activate employee assistance programs if needed.

MASS CASUALTY INCIDENTS (MCIs) are characterized by a rapid influx of patients that overwhelms the resources available in the ED, resulting in the activation of a contingency plan to bring more resources (staff, supplies, etc.) where they are needed. Examples of MCIs include mass shootings, sudden onset of contagious disease (e.g., flu season), MVCs involving buses or a large number of vehicles, train and airplane accidents, and biological/chemical accidents or attacks.

DECONTAMINATION must be performed by trained or certified individuals with a strong working knowledge of contaminants. Decontamination areas must be set up a good distance from any entrance into a hospital to avoid cross contamination of the area and building.

- The HOT ZONE of care is the point of entry to the decontamination process following an incident. Patients triaged as immediate, delayed, or nonambulatory will be decontaminated first. They are triaged in the hot zone and have their clothes removed as they approach the warm zone.

- The WARM ZONE is where active decontamination occurs. Decontamination usually includes the use of water, but this will depend on the chemical, biological, or radioactive agent the patient is exposed to.

- The COLD ZONE is the point of exit from the decontamination area. The patient enters the cold zone and may be treated onsite or transported to an appropriate level of care.

QUICK REVIEW QUESTION

17. What role does a nurse play in disaster management?

The Health Insurance Portability and Accountability Act (HIPAA)

The HEALTH INSURANCE PORTABILITY AND ACCOUNTABILITY ACT (HIPAA) requires that individual healthcare providers and healthcare organizations make

DID YOU KNOW?
A **pandemic** is an infectious disease that is prevalent on a global scale. An **epidemic** is an infectious disease that occurs in a community at a particular time, such as influenza.

DID YOU KNOW?
Natural disasters often result in widespread power outages, flooding, or structural damage that necessitate evacuation. All EDs must have a contingency plan for evacuation and support of patients requiring care following a large natural disaster.

every attempt to safeguard the **PROTECTED HEALTH INFORMATION (PHI)** of the patient. PHI is defined as any information that concerns the past, present, or future mental or physical health of the patient, along with the treatments of such health conditions and the methods of payment for health services rendered.

HIPAA is based on the **MINIMUM NECESSARY REQUIREMENT**; i.e., the minimum amount of PHI needed to accomplish a task should be shared. Sharing of PHI under HIPAA is permissible in the following contexts:

■ health care operations (e.g., care planning, quality improvement activities)

■ activities involving reimbursement or payment for care premiums, determining coverage or provision of benefits, etc.

■ competency assurance

■ audits of medical records for legal or competency reviews

■ insurance use

■ business planning, development, or management

■ public health reporting

■ fraud reporting

■ abuse and neglect reporting

■ organ and tissue donation

■ law enforcement proceedings

Many organizations employ HIPAA compliance officers in order to support both patients and the organization with compliance issues and training. If a patient believes their PHI was not protected appropriately, they should be referred to the compliance officer or the United States Department of Health and Human Services. Patients' rights under HIPAA include:

■ the right to receive information regarding how their PHI is used and protected

■ access to personal medical records (with some exceptions)

■ access to lists of nonroutine disclosures of their PHI

■ the right to dictate authorization to use their PHI and to restrict certain uses

QUICK REVIEW QUESTION

18. What should a nurse do when made aware of a possible HIPAA breach or violation?

Patient Consent for Treatment

Patient **CONSENT FOR TREATMENT** is a complex issue in the ED. Considerations include capacity for consent, age of consent, and state and federal laws governing when these considerations may be waived. In general, there are four types of consent: informed, implied, express, and involuntary.

DID YOU KNOW?
Sharing of PHI with patient's family or friends should only be done with the patient's explicit consent.

- **INFORMED CONSENT** is used in situations where moderately invasive or high-risk procedures are going to be performed. The provider must cover key elements for informed consent to be valid.
  - ☐ description of the procedure
  - ☐ risks and benefits of the procedure
  - ☐ alternative options available to the patient

- **IMPLIED CONSENT** is given in situations where patients are at risk to lose life or limb, and they are unable to provide informed consent. This type of consent is only applicable during resuscitation and is no longer implied if the patient is able to give and/or express informed consent.

- **EXPRESS CONSENT** is the assumption of consent to perform noninvasive to minimally invasive procedures in the ED. Some departments require a signature for express consent; others take verbal consent based on words or actions of patients.

- **INVOLUNTARY CONSENT** is given when a patient is deemed not to have decisional capacity. Physicians, law enforcement officers, and psychiatrists typically enact this type of consent.

PEDIATRIC CONSENT is another complex issue. If a pediatric patient presents for care without the presence of a legally responsible adult, the emergency nurse must get consent for care from the legal custodian of the patient. There are some exceptions to this rule:

- Treatment can be provided if there is immediate danger to life or limb.

- Some states allow pediatric patients to come to the ED for care of STIs or similar issues in the absence of the legal custodian.

- Treatment can be provided when there is high suspicion of non-accidental trauma or domestic abuse. Consent for treatment is implied until the local child services system can determine temporary legal guardianship terms.

QUICK REVIEW QUESTION

19. A 15-year-old male patient arrives at the ED requesting an evaluation for a possible STI. What kind of consent for treatment should be established?

Process Improvement

There are many opportunities to apply process improvement initiatives in the ED. The greatest opportunity for process improvement is in throughput and patient flow through the department, a task that nurses are largely responsible for managing. Measurement of metrics such as arrival to triage times, arrival to provider times, arrival to bed times, and arrival to disposition times can give excellent insight into process issues that can be addressed.

Process improvement projects normally follow structured programs such as Lean Six Sigma or 4DX in order to provide a framework to carry out the project. Generally, steps in process improvement include:

- identifying the problem
- measuring relevant variables for baseline metrics
- identifying, developing, and implementing a solution or change
- measuring the impact of the change

QUICK REVIEW QUESTION

20. The ED manager has noticed a steady increase in the percentage of patients leaving without being seen or leaving before being triaged. How should she investigate this problem?

Symptom Surveillance

HELPFUL HINT

Screening for infectious disease exposure typically occurs at triage through a series of questions about travel, recent social activities, or attendance at schools or churches.

In general, the emergency nurse is not required to recognize SYMPTOM CLUSTERS through sophisticated statistical methods such as spatial analysis. However, there is an obligation to report a concern of an acute influx of like symptoms within a community or population. Sources of infectious disease clustering may include:

- places where large numbers of people gather at a given time (e.g., schools, churches, concents, movie theaters, etc.)
- pediatric populations at schools or day cares
- foodborne illness can be spread through the distribution of food at grocery stores, restaurants, festivals, local farming co-ops, etc.

DID YOU KNOW?

Hospital systems have mechanisms to prompt mandatory disease reporting through ICD-10 coding, and generally do not require that individual practitioners submit such reports.

Disease surveillance is achieved through the systematic collection of data on certain MANDATORILY REPORTED DISEASES. There are many such diseases; those mostly commonly seen in the ED include:

- STIs
- viral diseases spread by mosquitos or other insect vectors
- chicken pox
- cholera
- all vaccine-preventable diseases

QUICK REVIEW QUESTION

21. An emergency nurse is on his third scheduled shift in a row, and he has noticed several pediatric patients presenting to the department with similar but vague symptoms. What should he do with this information?

TRIAGE

TRIAGE in the ED is defined as the method of sorting patients based on chief complaint, physical presentation, anticipated needed resources, and vital signs. There is not a universal triage system used in the United States. Some departments use the three-level triage system, categorizing patients as emergent, urgent, and nonurgent.

- **Emergent patients** require immediate care; condition is severe, and threat to life or limb is present.

- **Urgent patients** require care as soon as possible; condition is acute, and condition presents danger if not treated.

- **Nonurgent patients** can safely wait for care.

In many EDs, the **Emergency Severity Index (ESI)** is used as a triage algorithm to assign each patient with a level of acuity to assist with treatment priority decisions. The ESI has five levels of acuity.

- Level 5: This patient arrives at the department stable, and requires no resources as defined by ESI in order to address their chief complaint.

- Level 4: This patient arrives in stable condition and may require one resource to address the chief complaint.

- Level 3: This patient arrives in stable condition; however, two or more resources may be needed to care for the patient. This patient has the potential to deteriorate into a more acute state.

- Level 2: This patient is unstable and requires many resources to address care needs. The patient may deteriorate into needing immediate lifesaving intervention but does not require it immediately upon arrival.

- Level 1: This patient requires immediate life- or limb-saving intervention upon arrival.

The **triage nurse** in the ED requires a high level of skill and experience to determine, with limited information, the acuity of patients in an often chaotic and challenging environment. Triage nursing generally requires a formal orientation with clinical and didactic training. However, there are some red flags that all ED nurses should recognize as requiring immediate assessment or care:

- apnea
- choking
- irregular respiration patterns
- abnormally high/low respiratory or heart rate
- hypotension
- cyanosis
- altered LOC
- hypothermia or extreme fever
- severe pain

HELPFUL HINT

Immediate assessment and care is needed for any patient with a temperature > 104°F (40°C) or infants with a temperature > 100.4°F (38°C).

Quick Review Question

22. A patient approaches the triage desk to ask why patients who arrived later than him are being seen earlier. What is the best answer for this patient?

ANSWER KEY

1. Gather resources for the agency CISM, encourage her to use the resources, and assist her in a debriefing of the pediatric code if it was not already done.

2. Consider asking family if there is a living will or advance directive. If it is feasible, suggest an emergency meeting of the agency ethics committee if the two providers are unable to make a decision. Ultimately, the attending on record is responsible for the decision.

3. The nurse should not change practice or introduce new nursing interventions without a formal literature review and EBP change project. One article is not enough to support change in practice, and it should be a collaborative decision among the multidisciplinary team to make such changes.

4. Participate in any journal clubs available, meet with research coordinators, and join professional associations.

5. The nurse can produce a record of continuing education activities in the form of certificates or letters to credentialing offices or boards of nursing.

6. Emergency nurses can identify patient needs or gaps in care and can help the patient find resources to bridge the gap. In adult patients, the responsibility of the nurse ends once the resources are provided, presuming that the patient has the capacity to access the resources if they choose to.

7. The nurse should review the wishes of the patient and family regarding organ donation, contact the local procurement agency, and maintain the hemodynamic stability of the patient in preparation for organ procurement.

8. Continue to resuscitate the patient, and ask the daughter to procure the DNR paperwork, if it is available. Explain that the ED team cannot act on the request until it has been verified as a valid, legal document.

9. The nurse should describe the postmortem care procedures to the family in a sensitive manner. The nurse should take the opportunity to discuss things such as organ procurement (if appropriate) and give the family an opportunity to see the patient again. Offering CISM or grief support services to the family is appropriate.

10. The nurse should stop the technician in a professional manner and demonstrate proper evidence removal and collection to him. The nurse should not delay immediate life-saving measures but instead debrief with the technician after the incident to follow up on the feedback.

11. The nurse, in collaboration with the physician, can explain to the mother that general anesthesia is not needed to reduce her son's fractured arm, and doing it in the ED under moderate sedation greatly reduces both risks and time spent in the hospital.

12. The nurse manager should assist the nurse with reporting the incident through a patient safety reporting system, or the nurse manager should report it directly to the risk manager or quality management division of the agency. The nurse should anticipate the incident being investigated for formal root-cause analysis and provide as much detail as possible.

13. Patient satisfaction scores are the first step in identifying ways to improve the patient care experience and can also affect practice decisions. Patients often report issues they experience or witness that would otherwise go unreported. Measuring patient satisfaction contributes significantly to patient safety data.

14. The emergency nurse should make sure that the patient has adequate peripheral access and a catheter if appropriate, and should prepare the patient for flight, if applicable. The nurse should ensure that all consents for transfers are signed and in the patient's medical record.

15. The nurse can respectfully ask the patient if there is any religious consideration that he should be aware of as he begins to care for the patient. He should document these considerations in the medical record.

16. The nurse may ask the technician directly, ask the charge nurse, refer to local nursing policy, or ask the immediate supervisor or manager. She should not delegate the task without a definitive answer.

17. ED nurses must have a concrete understanding of their assigned role in a disaster, which may be different from their everyday role. Disaster management roles may involve START triage (at times outside of the actual department, at the casualty collection/delivery point), delayed treatment (management of patient triaged as yellow), patient movement and transport, decontamination (if trained), and palliative care for expectant patients.

18. The nurse should immediately report it to the HIPAA compliance office or to their immediate supervisor.

19. Due to the nature of the complaint, in some states it may be appropriate to take express consent. This patient is a pediatric patient by definition; however, the sensitivity of the complaint may preclude the need for parental consent.

20. The ED manager should consider the reasons patients are leaving, if that information is available. She should also monitor and assess other throughput metrics to determine if wait times are longer than normal or if there are other contributing factors. A process improvement project may be appropriate to address these issues.

21. He should communicate with the senior medical officer in the department or the public health representative to share these observations. He should not keep this information to himself, because it could quickly develop into a large public health concern.

22. The triage nurse should inform the patient of the triage system and explain that some patients may require rapid or immediate care, while others may not. The nurse should not lessen the importance of the patient's chief complaint but should instead explain that emergency care is not always provided on a first-come, first-served basis.

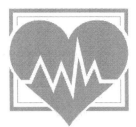

PRACTICE TEST

1. The ED nurse is caring for a patient with a subdural hematoma sustained in an automobile accident. The patient currently has an ICP of 22 mmHg. Which of the following would NOT be an appropriate intervention?

   A. BMP and CBC

   B. lumbar puncture

   C. mechanical ventilation

   D. Foley catheter placement

2. Which of the following substances is contraindicated for an 80-year-old patient with acute heart failure?

   A. dopamine

   B. adrenaline

   C. digoxin

   D. dobutamine

3. Which observation in a patient with abdominal aortic aneurysm indicates the need for immediate treatment?

   A. complaints of yellow-tinted vision

   B. hemoptysis

   C. urinary output of 75 mL/hr per urinary catheter

   D. complaints of sudden and severe back pain and dyspnea

4. The nurse is evaluating patients for risk of heparin-induced thrombocytopenia (HIT). Which patient is at greatest risk for HIT, based on the nurse's assessment?

   A. a male patient who just completed a 1-week course of heparin

   B. a male patient taking enoxaparin for management of unstable angina

   C. a female patient receiving heparin for postsurgical thromboprophylaxis

   D. a female patient taking enoxaparin to prevent clots following a mild myocardial infarction

5. During cardiac assessment of a patient with pericarditis, the nurse should expect to hear

   A. mitral regurgitation.

   B. S3 gallop.

   C. S4 gallop.

   D. pericardial friction rub.

6. Complications resulting from an untreated/ undertreated high-velocity injection injury may be minimized by

   A. educating the patient to return if signs of infection appear.

   B. administering prophylactic antibiotics.

   C. obtaining a surgical consultation and exploration.

   D. immobilizing the extremity involved.

7. A patient arrives in the ED with midsternal chest pain radiating down the left arm and left jaw. He slumps to the floor and is unresponsive, pulseless, and apneic. High-quality compressions are started, and the patient's ECG shows the following rhythm. What is the priority nursing intervention?

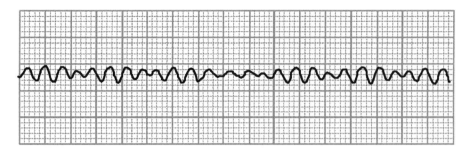

   A. administer a fluid bolus of 1 L normal saline
   B. defibrillate with 200 J
   C. administer 1 mg epinephrine IV
   D. insert an advanced airway

8. A patient comes to the ED complaining of intermittent nausea and vomiting for the past month. She states that she has pain in the abdomen that is relieved by eating. She began having diarrhea the day before. Medical history shows that the patient takes naproxen daily for arthritis. The nurse should assess for

   A. obesity.
   B. appendicitis.
   C. hypertension.
   D. gastritis.

9. An infant's parents bring him to the ED because of bloody, mucous stools. The child cries constantly and pulls his knees up to his chest. Which of the following findings would be the most critical?

   A. vomiting
   B. diarrhea
   C. abdominal swelling
   D. a lump in the abdomen

10. A patient with abdominal pain and possible appendicitis wants to leave the ED. What should the nurse do next?

   A. Inform the patient he will be involuntarily committed to the hospital if he tries to leave.
   B. Inform the physician of the patient's wish to leave.
   C. Warn the patient he will die if he leaves the department.
   D. Give the patient directions to the exit.

11. The current American Heart Association (AHA) guidelines for CPR on an adult patient with 2 rescuers is

   A. 30 compressions : 2 ventilations.
   B. 15 compressions : 2 ventilations.
   C. 30 compressions : 1 ventilation.
   D. 15 compressions : 1 ventilation.

12. A patient in the ED is diagnosed with a right ventricular infarction with hypotension. The nurse should prepare to administer which of the following to treat the hypotension?

   A. normal saline fluid boluses 1 to 2 L
   B. dopamine (Intropin) at 10 mcg/kg/min
   C. D5W fluid boluses titrate 3 L
   D. furosemide drip at 20 mg/hr

13. Which lab results confirm a diagnosis of carbon monoxide toxicity in a nonsmoking adult?

   A. COHb 0.8%
   B. COHb 8%
   C. $PaCO_2$ 38
   D. $PaCO_2$ 41

14. Which of the following procedures can be performed under procedural sedation in the ED?

   A. perimortem cesarean section
   B. synchronized cardioversion
   C. dilatation and curettage
   D. open fracture reduction

15. A 43-year-old female patient comes to the ED with complaints of vaginal discharge with itching and burning. The nurse notes a non-odorous white discharge that resembles cottage cheese. The nurse should prepare to treat the patient for which of the following?

    A. bacterial vaginosis

    B. trichomoniasis vaginitis

    C. Candida vulvovaginitis

    D. Neisseria gonorrhoeae

16. An 82-year-old patient presents to triage with a complaint of diarrhea for the past 3 days. She tells the triage nurse that she is on her third day of antibiotics. Which precautions should the nurse implement?

    A. airborne precautions

    B. contact precautions

    C. droplet precautions

    D. contact and droplet precautions

17. A 20-year-old female patient comes to the ED complaining of a green-gray frothy malodorous vaginal discharge and vaginal itching. The wet prep shows only WBCs. The nurse should prepare to assess for

    A. trichomoniasis.

    B. bacterial vaginosis.

    C. herpes simplex virus.

    D. chlamydia.

18. The nurse is performing an abdominal assessment on a patient with suspected heart failure. The patient asks the nurse the reason for assessing the abdomen. Which of the following would be the best response from the nurse?

    A. "Sometimes the medications used in heart failure will cause stomach upset."

    B. "Hepatomegaly, or an enlarged liver, is common in heart failure."

    C. "I am checking to see if you are constipated."

    D. "Heart failure can lead to appendicitis."

19. When trying to find a piece of glass in the soft tissue of the lateral thigh, which assessment technique should the nurse avoid?

    A. deep tissue palpation

    B. visual inspection

    C. palpation of distal pulses

    D. CSM of extremity

20. A patient who is 28 weeks pregnant presents to the ED with a malodorous vaginal discharge, a temperature of 102.3°F (39°C), and no complaints of uterine contractions. These signs and symptoms are most indicative of which of the following?

    A. septic spontaneous abortion

    B. ectopic pregnancy

    C. missed abortion

    D. abdominal trauma

21. A patient's cardiac monitor shows the rhythm below. He is awake and alert but is pale and confused. His blood pressure reads 64/40 mm Hg. What is the priority nursing intervention for this patient?

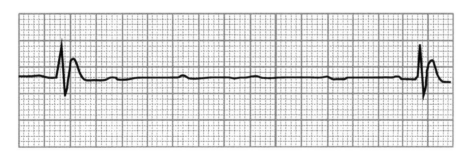

    A. defibrillate at 200 J

    B. prepare for transcutaneous pacing

    C. administer epinephrine 1 mg

    D. begin CPR

22.   The ECG in the exhibit supports the diagnosis of

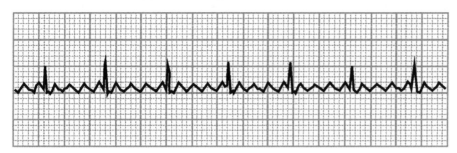

   A.   atrial flutter.
   B.   atrial fibrillation.
   C.   torsades de pointes.
   D.   ventricular fibrillation.

23.   Which of the following lab values should the nurse expect to order for a patient receiving IV heparin therapy for a pulmonary embolism?
   A.   hematocrit
   B.   HDL and LDL
   C.   PT and PTT
   D.   troponin level

24.   A patient is being treated for rapidly evolving disseminated intravascular coagulation (DIC) in the ED. Which of the following lab values would the nurse expect?
   A.   increased hemoglobin
   B.   decreased D-dimer
   C.   increased platelets
   D.   decreased fibrinogen

25.   The nurse is caring for a patient with Guillain–Barré syndrome who is at risk for autonomic dysfunction. The nurse should monitor the patient for
   A.   trigeminy.
   B.   heart block.
   C.   atrial flutter.
   D.   tachycardia.

26.   A nurse notes crackles while assessing lung sounds in a child with pneumonia. How would the nurse classify this respiratory disorder?
   A.   upper airway disorder
   B.   lower airway disorder
   C.   lung tissue disorder
   D.   disordered control of breathing

27.   A patient who was playing basketball outside all day has been drinking only water to stay hydrated. He suddenly became confused, complained of a headache, and collapsed. The nurse should suspect
   A.   hyperkalemia.
   B.   hyponatremia.
   C.   hypernatremia.
   D.   hypokalemia.

28.   Which of the following medications should a nurse anticipate administering to an 18-month-old patient with a barking cough first?
   A.   epinephrine 0.01 mg/kg IV stat
   B.   nebulized epinephrine breathing treatment
   C.   albuterol breathing treatment
   D.   dexamethasone PO or IV

29.   Classic signs of Bell's palsy include
   A.   facial droop, dysphagia, dysarthria.
   B.   facial droop, confusion, ataxia.
   C.   hemiparalysis, photophobia, headache.
   D.   tinnitus, nausea, vertigo.

30.   Which of the following is most likely to be found in a patient with left-sided heart failure?
   A.   jugular vein distention
   B.   crackles
   C.   hepatomegaly
   D.   ascites

31. Localized pain and edema associated with systemic fever and left shift differential may be indicative of

   A. foreign body infection of surgical hardware.

   B. superficial foreign body.

   C. buckle fracture.

   D. Achilles tendon rupture.

32. A 12-year-old patient is brought to the ED after falling 15 feet out of a tree. She is complaining of severe pain in the right side of the chest and severe dyspnea. Upon auscultation, the nurse notes absent breath sounds on the right and should suspect

   A. pneumothorax.

   B. foreign body lodged in the right side of the chest.

   C. hematoma.

   D. pleural effusion.

33. A patient with a subarachnoid hemorrhage from a fall at home arrives at the ED. When reviewing the medical orders, which medication order should prompt the nurse to notify the health care provider?

   A. warfarin

   B. morphine

   C. nimodipine

   D. a stool softener

34. Which symptom, identified by the patient, is the most common and consistent with a myocardial infarction?

   A. palpitations

   B. lower extremity edema

   C. feeling of pressure in the chest

   D. nausea

35. A patient arrives to the ED with a grossly deformed shoulder injury obtained while surfing. Suspecting a dislocation, which nursing intervention should the nurse initiate immediately?

   A. elevate the extremity

   B. put patient on NPO status

   C. apply ice

   D. provide ice chips

36. Which of the following statements should be included in the discharge instructions for a patient who has been prescribed carbamazepine to control seizures?

   A. Avoid exposure to sunlight.

   B. Limit foods high in vitamin K.

   C. Do not take on an empty stomach.

   D. Use caution when driving or operating machinery.

37. The nurse is caring for a patient with a traumatic brain injury who has a Glasgow Coma Scale (GCS) of 7. The nurse should anticipate the need to

   A. bolus with NS via IV.

   B. assist patient to chair.

   C. assist with intubation.

   D. apply 2L O_2 via nasal cannula.

38. The nurse is caring for a patient who just had a lumbar puncture to rule out meningitis. Which assessment finding would prompt the nurse to notify the health care provider?

   A. The patient is drinking fluids.

   B. The patient is lying flat in the bed.

   C. The patient's pain scale is 3 out of 10.

   D. The patient complains of severe headache.

39. A patient presents with signs and symptoms characteristic of myocardial infarction (MI). Which of the following diagnostic tools should the nurse anticipate will be used to determine the location of the myocardial damage?

   A. electrocardiogram

   B. echocardiogram

   C. cardiac enzymes

   D. cardiac catheterization

40. The ED nurse is waiting for a bed for a 72-year-old patient with Alzheimer's disease who has episodes of confusion. Which of the following will be included in the plan of care for this patient?

   A. prescribe haloperidol to prevent agitation

   B. provide toileting every 2 hours

   C. use restraints at night to prevent wandering

   D. allow choices when possible to promote feelings of respect

41. A 16-year-old patient arrives to the ED after ingesting an entire bottle of acetaminophen 4 hours before. The most appropriate intervention is

   A. administration of N-acetylcysteine.

   B. endotracheal intubation.

   C. administration of naloxone.

   D. gastric lavage.

42. A patient with emphysema comes to the ED complaining of dyspnea. The nurse should assist the patient into which of the following positions?

   A. lying flat on the back

   B. in a prone position

   C. sitting up and leaning forward

   D. lying on the side with feet elevated

43. A patient with severe dementia is brought to the ED for urinary retention. The patient repeatedly asks for her mother, who passed away many years ago. Which technique should the nurse use when the patient asks for her mother?

   A. confrontation

   B. reality orientation

   C. validation therapy

   D. seeking clarification

44. The nurse sees a bedbug on the personal linens of a child transported from the home setting to the ED via ambulance. What is the most appropriate action?

   A. Place the patient on airborne precautions.

   B. File a report with the local child welfare agency.

   C. Wash the patient thoroughly and replace all linens and clothing items with hospital-provided materials.

   D. Ask the parents to provide new clothing and linen from the home.

45. The nurse is caring for a patient with suspected diverticulitis. The nurse should anticipate all of the following findings EXCEPT

   A. fever.

   B. anorexia.

   C. lower abdominal pain.

   D. low WBC count.

46. A patient presents to the ED with abdominal pain and is found to have an incarcerated hernia. The patient is prepared for surgery. Which assessment finding by the nurse should be reported immediately to the health care provider?

   A. a burning sensation at the site of the hernia

   B. sudden nausea and vomiting with increased pain since arrival

   C. a palpable mass in the abdomen

   D. pain that occurs when bending over or coughing

47. EMS arrives to the ED with a stable adult patient who has a clear developmental delay. Emergent intervention is not needed upon arrival. What should the ED nurse do before treating the patient?

   A. Call the legal guardian of the patient to obtain consent for care.

   B. Continue to care for the patient.

   C. Obtain consent for care from the patient.

   D. Obtain permission from the hospital legal department to care for the patient.

48. A patient arrives at the ED complaining of severe pain to the right lower abdominal quadrant. The patient states that the pain is worse with coughing. The nursing assessment reveals that pain is relieved by bending the right hip. The patient has not had a bowel movement in three days. The nurse should anticipate all of the following interventions EXCEPT

   A. IV fluids.

   B. morphine 2mg IV.

   C. STAT MRI of abdomen.

   D. maintain NPO status.

49. A patient is admitted to the ED with an acute myocardial infarction (MI). The nurse is preparing the patient for transport to the cardiac catheterization laboratory. An alarm sounds on the cardiac monitor, and the patient becomes unresponsive. V-fib is noted. The nurse should anticipate doing which of the following first?

   A. beginning high-quality CPR

   B. defibrillation at 200 J

   C. administering epinephrine 1 mg

   D. placing an IV

50. A nursing home patient with an enterocutaneous fistula caused by an acute exacerbation of Crohn's disease arrives at the ED. The nursing priority is to

A. administer antibiotics.

B. preserve and protect the skin.

C. apply a wound VAC to the area.

D. provide quiet times for relaxation.

51. A patient with cardiogenic shock is expected to have

A. hypertension; dyspnea.

B. decreased urine output; warm, pink skin.

C. increased urine output; cool, clammy skin.

D. hypotension; weak pulse; cool, clammy skin.

52. A patient in the ED with chronic pain is requesting more intravenous pain medication for reported 10/10 pain. The physician will not give any more medication. How should the nurse approach this patient?

A. Inform the patient that it is the physician's decision.

B. Discuss chronic pain relief and realistic expectations with the patient.

C. Ignore the patient's pain complaint.

D. Discuss drug-seeking concerns with the patient.

53. Which appearance is most consistent with an avulsion?

A. open wound with presence of sloughing and eschar tissue

B. skin tear with approximated edges

C. shearing of the top epidermal layers

D. separation of skin from the underlying structures that cannot be approximated

54. The ED nurse receives a patient with blunt-force abdominal injury due to a knife wound. On inspection, a common kitchen knife is found in the patient's abdomen in the upper right quadrant. The patient is rapidly placed on a non-rebreather mask, two large-bore IVs are started, and labs are drawn. No evisceration is noted. Which should the nurse do next?

A. Notify next of kin.

B. Estimate blood loss.

C. Stabilize the knife with bulky dressings.

D. Attempt to gently pull the knife straight out.

55. In a hypothermic patient, hypovolemia occurs as the result of

A. diuresis and third spacing.

B. shivering and vasoconstriction.

C. diaphoresis and dehydration.

D. tachycardia and tachypnea.

56. A 14-year-old male patient is brought to the ED, stating he woke up in the middle of the night with sudden, severe groin pain and nausea. The pain persists despite elevation of the testes. These findings most likely indicate

A. testicular torsion.

B. epididymitis.

C. UTI.

D. orchitis.

57. A 16-year-old patient is brought to the ED complaining of abdominal pain, nausea, and sharp constant pain on both sides of the pelvis. She has a history of pelvic inflammatory disease and is not sexually active. The nurse notes a purulent vaginal discharge. These signs and symptoms are most indicative of which condition?

A. ectopic pregnancy

B. tubo-ovarian abscess

C. diverticulitis

D. ruptured appendix

58. A patient who is 9 weeks pregnant comes to the ED with complaints of abdominal cramping. During the physical assessment the nurse notes slight vaginal bleeding and a large, solid tissue clot. These findings most likely indicate

A. septic spontaneous abortion.

B. incomplete spontaneous abortion

C. threatened abortion.

D. complete spontaneous abortion.

59. A 4-month-old infant is brought to the ED with croup. Which of the following medications will the nurse administer in order to decrease inflammation?

A. ipratropium

B. albuterol

C. corticosteroids

D. antibiotics

60. The most common site of injection injuries is

   A. the second digit of the nondominant hand.

   B. the first digit of the nondominant hand.

   C. the second digit of the dominant hand.

   D. the first digit of the dominant hand.

61. A 21-year-old male patient reports to the ED with complaints of burning on urination and urethral itching. During the assessment, the nurse notes a mucopurulent discharge and no lesions. These signs and symptoms are most indicative of which of the following?

   A. chlamydia

   B. syphilis

   C. HPV

   D. herpes simplex virus

62. The mother of a 3-year-old patient diagnosed with varicella asks for the best at-home treatment. Which of the following treatments is NOT appropriate for the nurse to suggest?

   A. oral antihistamines

   B. colloidal oatmeal baths

   C. acetaminophen

   D. aspirin

63. A full-term neonate is delivered in the ED. After stimulation and suctioning, the infant is apneic with strong palpable pulses at 126/minute. The nursing priority is to

   A. rescue breaths at 12 – 20 breaths per minute.

   B. rescue breaths at 40 – 60 breaths per minute.

   C. insert endotracheal intubation.

   D. insert an LMA.

64. A pediatric patient in cardiopulmonary arrest has had a 40-minute resuscitation attempt in the ED. The ED nurse feels that the resuscitation is reaching the point of concern for medical futility. What is the nurse's responsibility at this time?

   A. Tell the parents to order the resuscitation attempt to be stopped.

   B. Suggest that the team leader consider ending the resuscitation.

   C. Order the team to stop the resuscitation.

   D. Continue with the resuscitation and allow the team leader to decide when to stop.

65. After an emergent delivery, a full-term infant is apneic with a pulse rate of 48 bpm. The infant has not responded to chest compressions. The nurse should prepare to administer

   A. atropine 0.5 mg/kg.

   B. epinephrine 0.01 – 0.03 mg/kg.

   C. sodium bicarbonate 1 to 2 mEq/mL.

   D. dobutamine drip.

66. Which treatment is appropriate for a minor blunt injury resulting in intact skin, ecchymosis, edema, and localized pain and tenderness?

   A. fasciotomy and opioid pain medications

   B. rest, ice, compression, elevation, and opioid pain medications

   C. rest, ice, compression, elevation, and use of NSAIDs

   D. immobilization and use of NSAIDs

67. A patient with depression and Alzheimer's disease presents to the ED complaining of abdominal pain. In reviewing the patient's health care orders, which medication should prompt the nurse to notify the health care provider?

   A. sertraline

   B. paroxetine

   C. memantine

   D. amitriptyline

68. A 14-year-old patient arrives to the ED with delirium, respiratory distress, and headache. Upon examination of the airway, the nurse notes a burn to the roof of the patient's mouth. What does the nurse suspect?

   A. ingestion of a hot beverage

   B. inhalation of chemicals from a compressed gas can

   C. ingestion of dry ice

   D. marijuana use

69. The nurse is caring for a patient who was brought to the ED with seizures. The patient begins having a seizure. The nursing priority is

   A. padding the bed rails.

   B. inserting a tongue blade.

   C. administering IV diazepam.

   D. turning the patient to his side.

70. A patient who is 32 weeks pregnant is having profuse bright red painless vaginal bleeding after being in a motor vehicle crash (MVC). The nurse should prepare to treat her for

   A. abruptio placentae.

   B. placenta previa.

   C. ectopic pregnancy.

   D. complete abortion.

71. A 30-week pregnant patient comes to the ED after falling down a flight of steps. She complains of uterine tenderness, and a small amount of dark bloody vaginal drainage is noted. The nurse should suspect

   A. abruptio placenta.

   B. placenta previa.

   C. incomplete spontaneous abortion.

   D. complete spontaneous abortion.

72. The ED nurse is caring for a patient with schizophrenia. The patient appears to be looking at someone and asks the nurse, "Aren't you going to speak to Martha?" No one else is in the room. Which response by the nurse is appropriate?

   A. "There's nobody there."

   B. "I will find a blanket for Martha."

   C. "Is Martha going to stay a while?"

   D. "Does Martha ever tell you to hurt yourself or others?"

73. A patient in the ED is having difficulty breathing and is diagnosed with a large plural effusion. The nurse prepares her for which of the following procedures?

   A. pericardiocentesis

   B. chest tube insertion

   C. thoracentesis

   D. pericardial window

74. When caring for a patient with esophageal varices, the nurse should first prepare to administer

   A. phenytoin

   B. octreotide

   C. levofloxacin

   D. pantoprazole

75. The ED nurse is caring for a patient who is deeply depressed following the death of her mother. She tells the nurse, "I just lost my world when Mom died. She was my anchor, and now I have no one." Which response by the nurse is the most appropriate?

   A. "You will feel better in time."

   B. "You should join a grief support group."

   C. "I felt the same way when my mother died."

   D. "You're feeling lost since your mother died."

76. A patient is admitted to the ED with chest pain. A 12-lead ECG is performed with ST elevations noted in leads II, III and aVF. The nurse should prepare to administer

   A. nitrates.

   B. diuretics.

   C. morphine.

   D. IV fluids.

77. A 20-year-old male college student arrives to the ED during spring break complaining of a headache, fever, nausea, and vomiting. He shows the ED nurse a petechial rash on his trunk and chest. Which of the following should the nurse suspect?

   A. influenza

   B. pertussis

   C. meningitis

   D. scabies

78. Epistaxis occurring from Kiesselbach's plexus is controlled by all methods EXCEPT

   A. cauterization of a visualized vessel.

   B. high Fowler's position leaning forward and applying continuous pressure to the midline septum.

   C. nasal packing with hemostatic material.

   D. endoscopic ligation.

79. Which of the following interventions is NOT appropriate for a patient with adrenal hypofunction?

   A. peripheral blood draws

   B. low-sodium diet

   C. blood glucose monitoring

   D. hydrocortisone therapy

80. A patient comes to the ED with complaints of nausea and vomiting for 3 days. His ECG reading is shown in the exhibit. The nurse should suspect

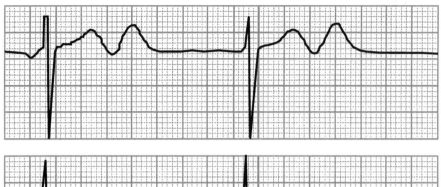
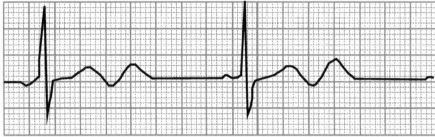

- **A.** hyperkalemia.
- **B.** hypokalemia.
- **C.** hypercalcemia.
- **D.** hypocalcemia.

81. An ED nurse is caring for a patient who was injured during a violent crime. Which of the following is a priority in evidence collection and care?

- **A.** chain of custody
- **B.** chain of evidence
- **C.** photographing of evidence
- **D.** documenting of evidence

82. A patient is brought to the ED following a motor vehicle crash. He was driving without a seat belt and was hit with the steering wheel on the left side of his chest. He complains of severe chest pain and dyspnea. During assessment, the nurse is unable to hear breath sounds on the left. The nurse should prepare to assist with immediate

- **A.** endotracheal intubation.
- **B.** chest compressions.
- **C.** chest tube insertion.
- **D.** thoracotomy.

83. A patient is brought to the ED with dyspnea, headache, light-headedness, and diaphoresis. A diagnosis of hyperventilation syndrome is made. The nurse is aware that hyperventilation syndrome can present with signs and symptoms similar to which of the following?

- **A.** pneumonia
- **B.** bronchitis
- **C.** pulmonary embolism
- **D.** pneumothorax

84. Which test should a nurse expect before a health care provider prescribes risperidone to manage psychotic symptoms?

- **A.** a cardiac workup
- **B.** comprehensive metabolic panel (CMP)
- **C.** creatinine clearance
- **D.** complete blood count (CBC)

85. The nurse is caring for a patient who says he wants to commit suicide. He has a detailed, concrete plan. The nurse places the patient on suicide precautions, which include a 24-hour sitter. The patient becomes angry and refuses the sitter. Which action is the most appropriate?

A. place the patient in soft wrist restraints

B. have security sit outside the patient's door

C. assign a sitter despite the patient's refusal

D. allow the patient to leave against medical advice (AMA)

86. Which laboratory finding indicates that a 62-year-old male patient is at risk for ventricular dysrhythmia?

A. magnesium 0.8 mEq/L

B. potassium 4.2 mmol/L

C. creatinine 1.3 mg/dL

D. total calcium 2.8 mmol/L

87. A patient presents to the ED with chest pain, dyspnea, and diaphoresis. The nurse finds a narrow complex tachycardia with a HR of 210 bpm, BP of 70/42 mm Hg, and a RR of 18. The nurse should anticipate which priority intervention?

A. administer adenosine 6 mg IV

B. defibrillate at 200 J

C. administer amiodarone 300 mg IV

D. prepare for synchronized cardioversion

88. A patient is brought to the ED in supraventricular tachycardia (SVT) with a rate of 220. EMS has administered 6 mg of adenosine, but the patient remains in SVT. What is the next intervention the nurse should anticipate?

A. administer 12 mg adenosine IV

B. administer 1 mg epinephrine IV

C. administer 300 mg amiodarone IV

D. administer 0.5 atropine IV

89. A patient is admitted to the ED with a sickle cell crisis. The nurse should prepare to administer which of the following blood products?

A. warm packed RBCs

B. whole blood

C. fresh frozen plasma (FFP)

D. cryoprecipitate

90. A 6-year-old child is admitted to the ED with an acute asthma attack. A pulse oximetry is attached with a reading of 91%. The nursing priority is to

A. administer dexamethasone.

B. provide supplemental oxygen.

C. prepare for immediate endotracheal intubation.

D. administer a nebulized albuterol treatment.

91. Which complication of compartment syndrome would the nurse suspect if urinalysis reveals myoglobinuria?

A. disseminated intravascular coagulation (DIC)

B. rhabdomyolysis

C. Volkmann's contracture

D. sepsis

92. A patient presents to the ED with complaints of substernal sharp, tearing knifelike chest pain radiating to the neck, jaw, and face. Morphine sulfate is given with no relief of the pain. These signs and symptoms are most indicative of which of the following?

A. myocardial infarction (MI)

B. pericarditis

C. pneumonia

D. acute aortic dissection

93. A patient is admitted to the ED with a potassium level of 6.9. Which of the following medications could have caused her electrolyte imbalance?

A. bumetanide

B. captopril

C. furosemide

D. digoxin

94. A patient presents to the ED with a bleeding laceration to the arm and a history of idiopathic thrombocytopenic purpura (ITP). The nurse should anticipate which treatment to be ordered?

A. cryoprecipitate

B. fresh frozen plasma (FFP)

C. platelets

D. protamine sulfate

95. Which of the following is usually associated with variant (Prinzmetal's) angina?

   A. cyanide poisoning

   B. gastroesophageal reflux

   C. Raynaud's phenomena

   D. beta-blocker toxicity

96. Hyperosmolar hyperglycemic state (HHS) is most often caused by

   A. inadequate glucose monitoring.

   B. dehydration.

   C. noncompliance with insulin therapy.

   D. a breakdown of ketones.

97. Fluoxetine for moderate depression is contraindicated in patients with

   A. arthritis.

   B. migraines.

   C. glaucoma.

   D. appendicitis.

98. A patient presents to the ED with severe throbbing fingers after coming home from the gym. Upon observing thin, shiny skin, pallor, and thick fingernails, the nurse should suspect

   A. acute arterial injury.

   B. acute arterial occlusion.

   C. peripheral venous thrombosis.

   D. peripheral vascular disease.

99. Which of the following IV solutions should be administered to a patient with diabetic ketoacidosis (DKA) who is placed on an insulin drip?

   A. lactated Ringer's

   B. normal saline

   C. normal saline with potassium

   D. normal saline with dextrose

100. When caring for a patient with thyroid storm, the nurse should first prepare to administer which medication?

   A. propylthiouracil (PTU)

   B. epinephrine

   C. levothyroxine

   D. atropine

101. EMS brings in a patient with a history of alcohol abuse, homelessness, and poor adherence to antiseizure medications. The patient has experienced 3 seizures in 30 minutes. These findings support the diagnosis of

   A. atonic seizure.

   B. tonic–clonic seizure.

   C. status epilepticus.

   D. simple partial seizure.

102. When taking the history of a patient with suspected pancreatitis, the nurse should expect to find

   A. the patient feels better when lying supine.

   B. the patient has a history of alcohol abuse and peptic ulcer disease.

   C. the pain is described as a sharp, burning sensation.

   D. the pain began gradually and radiated to the right lower abdomen.

103. A pediatric patient is being resuscitated in a trauma bay, and his father wants to be in the room. What should the nurse do?

   A. Tell the father he may not be in the trauma room during resuscitation.

   B. Allow the father in the trauma room with a knowledgeable staff member for support.

   C. Ask the father to stand just outside the trauma room.

   D. Call the legal department for advice.

104. A patient arrives to the ED after an attempted suicide by a self-inflicted gunshot wound. He is determined to be brain dead, but his life can be sustained for organ procurement. The patient is identified as an organ donor. Which of the following is the next step for the ED nurse?

   A. notify local organ procurement organization

   B. remove all life-supporting interventions

   C. perform postmortem care on the patient

   D. complete the death certificate

105. Which of the following signs or symptoms should lead a nurse to suspect septic shock?

   A. WBC of 2,500

   B. serum lactate level of 2.6

   C. decrease in neutrophils

   D. increase in RBCs

106. A patient arrives to the ED with a sheriff escort after being found in a street acting erratically and shouting. She is unkempt and not appropriately dressed for the weather. She states that she wants to commit suicide. What can the ED nurse expect to happen to the patient?

   A. She will be given benzodiazepines for anxiety and discharged.

   B. She will be medically cleared and brought to jail.

   C. She will be involuntarily committed.

   D. She will be voluntarily admitted to the hospital.

107. A patient with a blood glucose reading of 475 mg/dL presents to the ED with Kussmaul respirations, nausea, and vomiting, and a pH of 7.3. The nurse should expect to treat which condition?

   A. myxedema coma

   B. hyperosmolar hyperglycemic state (HHS)

   C. pheochromocytoma

   D. diabetic ketoacidosis (DKA)

108. The nurse is using the Glasgow Coma Scale (GCS) to assess a patient who fell in a parking lot. The patient opens his eyes to sound, localizes pain, and makes incoherent sounds when spoken to. Which GCS score will the nurse document?

   A. 9

   B. 10

   C. 11

   D. 12

109. A patient arrives to the ED with a complaint of sore throat and fever. Which of the following findings is the most immediate concern?

   A. visualized white abscess on the soft palate

   B. patchy tonsillar exudate

   C. petechiae on the hard palate

   D. lymphedema

110. A patient in the ED is diagnosed with ulcerative colitis (UC). Which dietary changes can the nurse recommend to help manage symptoms?

   A. Eat a high-fiber diet.

   B. Limit coffee to two cups daily.

   C. Avoid lactose-containing foods.

   D. Consume dried fruit several times a week.

111. A 32-year-old female patient comes to the ED with complaints of abdominal pain. She describes the pain as sharp and states it began suddenly during intercourse. The pain is worse with movement, and there is no vaginal discharge noted. These findings support the diagnosis of

   A. ectopic pregnancy.

   B. ruptured appendix.

   C. ruptured ovarian cyst.

   D. STD.

112. A patient is admitted to the ED with nausea, vomiting, and diarrhea for 3 days and signs of severe dehydration. The nurse starts an IV and prepares to administer which fluid replacement?

   A. hypertonic solution

   B. isotonic crystalloid

   C. hypotonic solution

   D. colloid solution

113. The nurse is reviewing the history of a patient with heart failure. Which of the following coexisting health problems will cause an increase in the patient's afterload?

   A. diabetes

   B. endocrine disorders

   C. hypertension

   D. Marfan syndrome

114. The nurse is caring for a patient who presented to the ED with a subarachnoid hemorrhage. While taking the patient's history, what symptoms would the nurse expect to see with this patient?

   A. sudden food cravings

   B. rash on the lower trunk

   C. Battle's sign

   D. a severe, sudden headache

115. Lower abdominal pain that is worsened with movement, a non-malodorous vaginal discharge, a fever, and tachycardia are usually associated with

   A. appendicitis.

   B. pelvic inflammatory disease.

   C. ectopic pregnancy.

   D. STI.

116. The nurse is discharging a patient who has been prescribed medications to control progressive MS. Which statement by the patient indicates a need for further teaching by the nurse?

   A. "I will wear an eye patch on alternating eyes if I have double vision."

   B. "I will clear rugs and extra furniture from my walking paths at home."

   C. "I hope I feel like going to Disney World this summer with my grandchildren."

   D. "I will call my doctor if I have any signs or symptoms of infection, such as fever."

117. Which prescription would the nurse anticipate administering to a patient with no known medication allergies who presents with orofacial edema, halitosis, and a complaint of tasting pus in the mouth?

   A. nystatin

   B. sodium fluoride drops

   C. penicillin V potassium

   D. saliva substitute

118. A patient with a myocardial infarction (MI) presents to the ED. The patient has received nitroglycerin sublingual and is still experiencing chest pain. The nurse should prepare to administer

   A. hydromorphone.

   B. meperidine.

   C. morphine sulfate.

   D. acetaminophen.

119. A patient presents to the ED with complaints of dizziness and fatigue and a past medical history of HIV. She states she is noncompliant with her antiviral medications. Her temperature is 101.2°F (38.4°C), BP 100/72 mm Hg, HR 130 bpm, RR 22, and O$_2$ 96%.

   Which of the following orders would be the priority intervention?

   A. administering an antibiotic

   B. administering acetaminophen

   C. administering prescribed antivirals

   D. administering 2 units of packed RBCs

120. The nurse is caring for a patient who suffered a head injury following a fall off a ladder. The nurse assesses the patient for signs of increased intracranial pressure (ICP). Which finding by the nurse is a LATE sign of increased ICP?

   A. headache

   B. restlessness

   C. dilated pupils

   D. decreasing LOC

121. An 11-month-old infant is brought to the ED with a barking cough, a respiratory rate of 66, substernal retractions, and copious nasal secretions. Which of the following positions will best facilitate the child's breathing?

   A. sitting upright in a parent's lap

   B. on a stretcher in a prone position

   C. reverse Trendelenburg

   D. semi-Fowler's

122. Which of the following statements would be included in the discharge teaching for a patient with ulcerative colitis (UC)?

   A. "Hemorrhage is a potential complication."

   B. "Patients may have 5 – 6 loose stools per day."

   C. "Patients with UC are more likely to have fistulas."

   D. "Many times, surgery is needed to treat symptoms."

123. Which pain characteristics are associated with inflammation of the fifth cranial nerve?

   A. progressive onset, bilateral, throbbing

   B. abrupt onset, unilateral, hemifacial spasm

   C. intermittent, circumoral, shooting

   D. paroxysmal, bilateral, paresthesia

124. Two weeks post–left-sided myocardial infarction (MI) a patient presents to the ED with dyspnea and cough with hemoptysis. The nurse should suspect the patient has developed

   A. pneumonia.

   B. over-coagulation.

   C. pulmonary edema.

   D. ruptured ventricle.

125. A patient arrives to the ED with altered mental status, blood pressure of 70/40, and declining vital signs. Her husband states that she does not wish to be resuscitated. What should the ED nurse do?

A. Tell the patient that the physician will decide her advance directive status.

B. Ask the spouse for the advance directive paperwork.

C. Document the patient's advance directive wishes and honor the request in case resuscitation is needed.

D. Inform the patient that advance directives are not used in EDs.

126. A family in the ED must decide whether to withdraw care for a family member with no advance directive. Which person would NOT be consulted as a part of a multidisciplinary team to make this decision?

A. chair of ethics committee

B. legal department

C. critical care physician

D. pharmacist

127. A 2-year-old child presents to the ED with septal deviation and a visualized foreign body in the right naris. Which nursing intervention is most appropriate?

A. instructing the parent to perform nasal positive pressure

B. instructing the child to blow his nose

C. instructing the parent to perform oral positive pressure

D. restraining the child for forceps retraction

128. The nurse is caring for a patient with a history of cirrhosis who arrived at the ED with a new onset of confusion. The patient's skin is jaundiced. Labs are as follows:

Ammonia 130 mcg/dL

ALT 98 U/L

Blood glucose 128

The nurse should prepare to administer

A. lactulose.

B. bisacodyl.

C. mesalamine.

D. insulin 2 units.

129. Which treatment is contraindicated for a corneal abrasion?

A. application of ophthalmic lubricating solution

B. application of topical anesthetics

C. patching the affected eye

D. wearing glasses instead of contact lenses

130. The ED nurse is caring for a patient with delirium who tells the nurse, "There are snakes crawling up on my bed." How should the nurse respond?

A. "That's just the wrinkles in your blanket."

B. "I will see if I can move you to another room."

C. "I will call maintenance to come and remove them."

D. "I know you're scared, but I don't see any snakes on your bed."

131. The nurse is caring for a patient who has been prescribed rasagiline mesylate for Parkinson's disease. Which medication on the patient's current record should prompt the nurse to notify the health care provider?

A. baclofen

B. amantadine

C. benztropine

D. isocarboxazid

132. Which medication would the nurse anticipate administering to a patient with a periorbital vesicular rash along the trigeminal nerve?

A. acyclovir

B. erythromycin

C. ketorolac

D. ciprofloxacin

133. Discharge teaching for a patient diagnosed with ulcerative keratitis is effective if she states which of the following?

A. "There is no need to follow up with an ophthalmologist."

B. "I will stop the antibiotic drops tomorrow if the pain is better."

C. "I will wear glasses and not contacts for at least two weeks."

D. "I need to stay home from work until the infection clears because I am highly contagious."

134. The nurse is caring for a patient who presents to the ED with the following arterial blood gas (ABG) results:

pH 7.32

$PaCO_2$ 47 mm Hg

HCO_3 24 mEq/L

PaO_2 91 mm Hg

The nurse should expect the patient to present with

A. chest pain.

B. nausea and vomiting.

C. deep, rapid respirations.

D. hypoventilation with hypoxia.

135. Management of acute iritis includes

A. topical mydriatic ophthalmic drops and topical corticosteroids.

B. copious irrigation.

C. IV mannitol and acetazolamide.

D. topical anesthetics and topical antibiotics.

136. Which of the following is a clinical feature of an open globe rupture?

A. cherry red macula

B. rust ring

C. pale optic disc

D. afferent pupillary defect

137. Which statement regarding tourniquet use to control hemorrhagic bleeding for a partial limb amputation is correct?

A. A commercially available tourniquet that is at least 2 inches wide with a windlass, a ratcheting device to occlude arterial flow, is recommended.

B. Tourniquet application is never recommended even when direct pressure does not control blood loss from an extremity.

C. Tourniquets properly applied in the prehospital setting should always be removed upon arrival to the ED, regardless if there is adequate team support to manage bleeding.

D. Time of tourniquet application should be noted clearly on the device and should not exceed 4-hour intervals before reassessment of bleeding.

138. Dopamine (Intropin) is ordered for a patient with heart failure because the drug

A. lowers the heart rate.

B. opens blocked arteries.

C. prevents plaque from building up.

D. increases the amount of oxygen delivered to the heart.

139. Which of the following will confirm the diagnosis of a pulmonary embolism?

A. chest X-ray

B. D-dimer

C. fibrin split products

D. CT angiography

140. The nurse is caring for a patient with a history of schizophrenia, alcohol abuse, bipolar disorder, and noncompliance with treatment and medications. The patient has also been arrested in the past for violent behavior. Which action by the nurse is the most important when caring for a potentially violent patient?

A. treat the patient with courtesy and respect

B. always maintain an open pathway to the door

C. be sure the patient swallows his pills and does not "cheek" them

D. ask permission from the patient before drawing blood or performing other invasive procedures

141. A 13-year-old female arrives to the ED complaining of chest pain. A physical exam reveals tenderness along the fourth, fifth, and sixth ribs. Which diagnosis does the nurse suspect?

A. myocardial infarction

B. Ludwig's angina

C. pleurisy

D. costochondritis

142. Diagnostic findings common with gouty arthritis include

A. hyperammonemia.

B. hyperbilirubinemia.

C. hyperuricemia.

D. hyperhomocysteinemia.

143. Which of the following describes the characteristics of a flail chest?

    A. The chest sinks in with inspiration and out with expiration.

    B. Only the right side of the chest has movement.

    C. Movement is noted on the left side of the chest only.

    D. There is no movement noted on either side of the chest.

144. A 4-year-old child was in a bicycle accident and presents with oral lacerations and complete dental avulsions to the 2 top front teeth. The best initial management by the health care provider is

    A. immediate replantation of the avulsed teeth.

    B. laceration repair.

    C. replantation of the avulsed tooth after soaking for 30 minutes in Hank's solution.

    D. dental consult.

145. Which dressing would be most appropriate for a patient with a partial thickness wound to the epidermis?

    A. transparent dressing

    B. occlusive dressing

    C. nonstick adherent dressing

    D. bulky dressing

146. A patient arrives to the ED from a house fire. The nurse notes soot at the opening of her mouth and both nares. What is the primary concern for this patient?

    A. total body surface areas covered in burns

    B. airway edema related to inhalation injury

    C. foreign body ingestion during the fire

    D. trauma as a result of rescue from the fire

147. Which intervention is contraindicated for a patient with acute angle glaucoma?

    A. administration of ophthalmic beta blocker

    B. maintaining patient in a supine position

    C. dimming lights in the room or providing a blindfold for comfort

    D. administration of IV mannitol

148. The ED nurse is providing discharge teaching to a patient newly diagnosed with migraines who has been given a prescription for sumatriptan. Which of the following statements indicates the patient understands the discharge teaching?

    A. "This medication is safe to take while pregnant."

    B. "I will report chest pain immediately to my physician."

    C. "I will take my blood pressure medicine before I take sumatriptan."

    D. "I will take this medication 15 minutes after I feel a migraine starting."

149. Which of the following chest X-ray readings is consistent with acute respiratory distress syndrome (ARDS)?

    A. bilateral, diffuse white infiltrates without cardiomegaly

    B. bilateral, diffuse infiltrates with cardiomegaly

    C. tapering vascular shadows with hyperlucency and right ventricular enlargement

    D. prominent hilar vascular shadows with left ventricular enlargement

150. Which positive toxicology result would the nurse suspect in a patient with a MRSA-positive infectious abscess of the right antecubital space?

    A. alcohol

    B. opioid

    C. benzodiazepine

    D. tetrahydrocannabinol (THC)

151. A patient arrives to the ED after taking a sedative and subsequently becoming confused and disoriented. His temperature is 96.2°F (35.6°C), pulse is 47 bpm with distant heart tones, and BP is 82/65 mm Hg. He states that he is currently receiving thyroid replacement therapy. The nurse should suspect

    A. allergic reaction to the sedative.

    B. thyroid storm.

    C. myxedema coma.

    D. acute stroke.

152. The health care provider orders xylocaine with epinephrine to be prepared for a patient with a

  A. 2 cm laceration to the penile shaft.

  B. 2 cm laceration above the right eyebrow.

  C. 3 cm laceration to the left index finger.

  D. 7 cm laceration to the left forearm.

153. Which is the most appropriate post-exposure rabies prophylaxis treatment for an animal bite in a patient not previously vaccinated?

  A. rabies vaccine on days 0, 3, 7, and 14

  B. human rabies immune globulin injected into the wound bed

  C. human rabies immune globulin injected into the wound bed and rabies vaccine on days 0, 3, 7, and 14

  D. tetanus 0.5 mL via intramuscular injection

154. A child is admitted to the ED with wheezing on exhalation, use of accessory muscles, using 1-word sentences, and tripod positioning. The nurse should suspect

  A. pneumonia.

  B. pneumonitis.

  C. foreign body aspiration.

  D. asthma.

155. Which of the following IV medications should a nurse anticipate administering to a patient experiencing a severe anaphylactic reaction to a bee sting?

  A. epinephrine 1:1000 0.3 – 0.5 mL

  B. diphenhydramine 25 – 50 mg

  C. Solu-Medrol 125 mg

  D. theophylline 6mg/kg

156. The best medical management for carbon monoxide toxicity is

  A. hydroxocobalamin

  B. hyperbaric oxygen

  C. N-acetylcysteine

  D. sodium bicarbonate

157. A patient presents to the ED with complaints of severe headache, irritability, confusion, and lethargy. During triage he mentions that he has spent the last several days in his shop with a wood-burning stove. The ED nurse should be concerned for which of the following?

  A. migraine headache

  B. stroke

  C. carbon monoxide poisoning

  D. allergic reaction

158. The nurse is reviewing the laboratory results of a patient with renal failure and notes a serum potassium level of 7.2. The nurse should prepare to administer which of the following medications to protect cardiac status?

  A. aspirin

  B. insulin

  C. calcium gluconate

  D. digoxin

159. A college student arrived at the ED with suspected meningitis, and a positive diagnosis was confirmed via lumbar puncture. Which of the following findings suggests that she may have developed hydrocephalus?

  A. sluggish pupillary response

  B. inability to wrinkle the forehead

  C. inability to move the eyes laterally

  D. inability to move the eyes downward

160. Appropriate discharge teaching for a patient with diverticular disease includes instructions to

  A. avoid foods high in sodium.

  B. consume clear liquids until pain subsides.

  C. limit alcohol to one glass per day.

  D. include strawberries to get enough vitamin C.

161. Which neurological assessment finding commonly occurs in a patient struck by lightning?

  A. tic douloureux

  B. ascending paralysis

  C. Bell's palsy

  D. keraunoparalysis

162. A patient presents to the ED with confusion, anxiety, irritability, and a slight tremor. During assessment, she states she drinks two or more bottles of wine per day. Which of the following questions is important to ask?

   A. Do you drink any other alcoholic drinks on a regular basis?

   B. When was your last drink?

   C. When was your first drink?

   D. Have you ever experienced alcohol withdrawal?

163. A 34-year-old patient attempted suicide by consuming his grandmother's oral antidiabetic agent. Administration of glucose has been unsuccessful in reversing the effect of the medication. Which antidote should the nurse expect to administer next?

   A. flumazenil

   B. acetylcysteine

   C. octreotide

   D. methylene blue

164. A patient presents to triage with a complaint of cough lasting three weeks without improvement. The patient confirms recent travel to a developing country, and states she has had fevers and chills for the last three days. The nurse should suspect

   A. herpes zoster.

   B. tuberculosis.

   C. influenza.

   D. hepatitis C.

165. A woman arrives to the ED with her 5-year-old child, whom she discovered eating her nifedipine. She does not know how many pills the child consumed. The nursing priority is to

   A. place a referral to child protective services.

   B. obtain a 12-lead ECG.

   C. place the child on oxygen.

   D. ask the child how many she took.

166. Which of the following medications should the nurse expect to administer to a patient who chronically abuses alcohol?

   A. naloxone

   B. thiamine

   C. flumazenil

   D. vitamin K

167. A 10-year-old child presents to triage with conjunctivitis, cough, and a rash in the back of his mouth. During the assessment, the patient's father indicates that the child is not vaccinated. These findings most likely indicate

   A. varicella.

   B. mumps.

   C. measles.

   D. pertussis.

168. A 35-year-old patient in the ED has been diagnosed with herpes zoster. Which of the following statements should the nurse include in her discharge teaching?

   A. Herpes zoster occurs any time after an initial varicella infection and may recur several times.

   B. The varicella vaccine is known to cause latent herpes zoster when administered to children.

   C. Herpes zoster outbreaks are caused by a latent virus, so it is not contagious.

   D. The zoster vaccine should not be given to patients who have had a herpes zoster outbreak.

169. A 7-year-old unvaccinated child arrives to the ED. The nurse suspects diphtheria, based on which of the following symptoms?

   A. thick gray membrane covering the tonsils and pharynx

   B. temperature of 104°F (40°C) or greater

   C. macular rash on the thorax and back, along the dermatomes

   D. cluster headache with nausea and symptoms of an aura

170. Which of the following statements from a nurse demonstrates that his participation in a Critical Incident Stress Debriefing (CISD) session was effective?

   A. He agrees to meet with the manager regarding the incident.

   B. He agrees to attend future debriefing sessions as needed.

   C. He agrees to schedule an appointment for further counseling.

   D. He provides the incident details before departing the debrief.

171. The ED nurse's responsibility to practice quality nursing care is achieved through which of the following?

    A.   reading research articles

    B.   participating in Evidence-Based Practice (EBP) projects

    C.   participating in research studies

    D.   participating in grand rounds

172. Nurses managing patient transitions of care in the ED should consider all of the following characteristics EXCEPT

    A.   accessibility of services.

    B.   safety.

    C.   community partnerships.

    D.   patient income.

173. What is the appropriate ratio of compressions to ventilations for a full-term neonate who is apneic with a pulse rate of 50 bpm?

    A.   30:2

    B.   15:1

    C.   15:2

    D.   3:1

174. Which of the following interventions is NOT necessary for a patient who has died in the ED and is not in a vegetative state?

    A.   maintaining the head of the bed at 20 degrees

    B.   instilling artificial tears in eyes to preserve tissue

    C.   taping eyes closed with paper tape

    D.   inserting Foley catheter to decompress the bladder

175. A 24-year-old male patient arrives at the ED with a complaint of a 1-month history of a rash that is annular, with raised margins and centralized clearing. Which of the following dermal infections does the nurse expect?

    A.   scabies

    B.   ringworm

    C.   impetigo

    D.   cellulitis

ANSWER KEY

1. B.

Rationale: Lumbar punctures are contraindicated for patients with increased ICP because of the risk of brain shift caused by the sudden release of CSF pressure. Severe brain shift can result in permanent damage. BMP and CBC labs are routinely monitored in patients with increased ICP. Mechanical ventilation and Foley catheter placement are commonly ordered for patients with increased ICP.

Objective: Neurological Emergencies

Subobjective: Increased Intracranial Pressure (ICP)

2. C.

Rationale: Adrenaline, dopamine, digoxin, and dobutamine are all positive inotropes and can be helpful in the management of heart failure. However, digoxin is not recommended in the treatment of acute heart failure in an 80-year-old patient as elderly patients are more susceptible to digoxin toxicity.

Objective: Cardiovascular Emergencies

Subobjective: Heart Failure

3. D.

Rationale: Sudden back pain and dyspnea indicate rupture of the aneurysm, which is an emergency. The nurse should notify the health care provider, monitor neurological and vital signs, and remain with the patient. Yellow-tinted vision is a finding of digitalis toxicity. Hemoptysis a sign of pulmonary edema. Urinary output of 75 mL/hr is normal.

Objective: Cardiovascular Emergencies

Subobjective: Aneurysm/Dissection

4. C.

Rationale: Increased risk factors for heparin-induced thrombocytopenia (HIT) include being female and heparin use for postsurgical thromboprophylaxis. HIT is more common in patients who have been on unfractionated heparin or who have used heparin for longer than 1 week. Enoxaparin is a low-molecular-weight heparin, which carries a lower risk of causing HIT. It is often prescribed for patients with unstable angina to help increase blood flow through the heart.

Objective: Cardiovascular Emergencies

Subobjective: Thromboembolic Disease

5. D.

Rationale: A pericardial friction rub is heard in pericarditis due to the inflammation of the pericardial layers rubbing together. Mitral regurgitation does not occur in pericarditis. An S3 gallop is heard in heart failure. S4 gallop is heard in cardiomyopathies and congenital heart disease.

Objective: Cardiovascular Emergencies

Subobjective: Pericarditis

6. C.

Rationale: High-velocity injection injuries damage underlying tissue and often result in necrosis and compartment syndrome and may require amputation. Obtaining a surgical consultation and exploration minimizes the risk of long-term complications. While administering prophylactic antibiotics, providing patient education, and immobilizing the affected extremity are correct nursing interventions, they alone will not minimize the risk for complications.

Objective: Wound

Subobjective: Injection Injuries

7. B.

Rationale: The patient is in V-fib and is pulseless. After CPR is started, the next priority intervention is defibrillation. Epinephrine should not be administered until after defibrillation. Inserting an advanced airway may be indicated but is not the priority. A fluid bolus is not a priority for a patient in V-fib.

Objective: Cardiovascular Emergencies

Subobjective: Cardiopulmonary Arrest

8. D.

Rationale: The patient has signs and symptoms of gastritis. Pain relievers such as naproxen can inflame the lining of the stomach and lead to gastritis. Tobacco use, radiation, and viral or bacterial infection are also risk factors. Obesity, appendicitis, and hypertension are not associated with naproxen.

Objective: Gastrointestinal Emergencies

Subobjective: Gastritis

9. C.

Rationale: The infant has signs of intussusception, in which part of the intestine telescopes into another area of the intestine. Abdominal swelling in a child with intussusception is a sign of peritonitis, which can be life-threatening. Vomiting, diarrhea, and a lump in the abdomen are expected findings in a child with intussusception.

Objective: Gastrointestinal Emergencies

Subobjective: Intussusception

10. **B.**

Rationale: The physician will counsel the patient on the risks associated with leaving against medical advice (AMA). Whenever possible, the patient should be counseled by the physician, sign AMA paperwork, and then leave the department. A patient with appendicitis will not be involuntarily committed. It is not appropriate to tell a patient he will die if he leaves, although he should be informed of possible negative consequences. The patient should speak with the physician before he tries to leave.

Objective: Professional Issues

Subobjective: Patient (Discharge Planning)

11. **A.**

Rationale: Current 2015 guidelines for CPR from the AHA is 30 compressions to 2 ventilations for adult patients with 2 rescuers.

Objective: Cardiovascular Emergencies

Subobjective: Cardiopulmonary Arrest

12. **A.**

Rationale: Fluid boluses of 1 to 2 L normal saline should be used to treat hypotension. The patient is dehydrated at the cellular level and needs fluid resuscitation. Furosemide is used as a diuretic and would further dehydrate the patient, exacerbating the issue. Inotropes such as dopamine are used to promote cardiac contractility and will not hydrate the patient. D5W is not indicated because it is not an isotonic solution that will add to the systemic fluid volume.

Objective: Cardiac Emergencies

Subobjective: Acute Coronary Syndromes

13. **B.**

Rationale: An elevated carboxyhemoglobin (COHb) level of 2% or higher for nonsmokers and 10% or higher for smokers strongly supports a diagnosis of carbon monoxide poisoning. COHb may be measured with a fingertip pulse

CO-oximeter or by serum lab values. $PaCO_2$ measurements remain normal (38 – 42).

Objective: Environmental

Subobjective: Chemical Exposure

14. **B.**

Rationale: Procedural sedation is appropriate for synchronized cardioversion. A perimortem cesarean section typically is done emergently. Open fracture reductions should occur in the operating room, as should dilatation and curettage.

Objective: Professional Issues

Subobjective: Patient (Pain Management and Procedural Sedation)

15. **C.**

Rationale: A non-odorous white "cottage cheese"–appearing vaginal discharge describes Candida vulvovaginitis. Bacterial vaginosis presents with thin white, gray, or green discharge and a fishy odor. Trichomoniasis vaginitis typically presents with thin discharge and itching or burning of the genital area. Neisseria gonorrhoeae usually does not cause any symptoms but may have dysuria and thin discharge.

Objective: Gynecological

Subobjective: Infection

16. **B.**

Rationale: The nurse should place the patient on contact precautions with concern for *C. difficile*. The other levels of precautions are not appropriate based on the information presented.

Objective: Communicable Diseases

Subobjective: C. Difficile

17. **A.**

Rationale: A greenish-gray frothy malodorous vaginal discharge and itching are signs and symptoms of trichomoniasis. Bacterial vaginosis would present with a thin discharge and presence of clue cells on the wet prep. Herpes would most likely present with lesions upon inspection. Chlamydia would not cause frothy discharge.

Objective: Gynecological

Subobjective: Infection

18. **B.**

Rationale: Hepatomegaly is seen in patients with right-sided heart failure due to vascular engorgement. Heart failure does not lead to appendicitis. Constipation is not directly a result of heart failure and therefore is not a priority assessment consideration. Stomach upset is a common side effect of many medications but is not a cause for focused or priority assessment.

Objective: Cardiac Emergencies

Subobjective: Heart Failure

19. **A.**

Rationale: Deep tissue palpation should be avoided to minimize the risk of injury to the nurse and to prevent advancement of the foreign body deeper into the tissue structure.

Objective: Wound

Subobjective: Foreign Bodies

20. **A.**

Rationale: The patient's symptoms are signs of a septic abortion. An ectopic pregnancy typically presents with vaginal bleeding and pain without fever. A missed abortion may have no other symptoms except a brown discharge. The symptoms are not indicative of abdominal trauma.

Objective: Obstetrical

Subobjective: Threatened/Spontaneous Abortion

21. **B.**

Rationale: The patient is unstable in a third-degree or complete heart block, so transcutaneous pacing is indicated.

Objective: Cardiovascular Emergencies

Subobjective: Dysrhythmias

22. **A.**

Rationale: In atrial flutter, there are no discernible P waves, and a distinct sawtooth wave pattern is present. The atrial rate is regular, and the PR interval is not measurable. In atrial fibrillation, the rhythm would be very irregular with coarse, asynchronous waves. Torsades de pointes, or "twisting of the points," is characterized by QRS complexes that twist around the baseline and is a form of polymorphic ventricular tachycardia. It may resolve spontaneously or progress to ventricular fibrillation, which is emergent, as the ventricles are unable to pump any blood due to disorganized electrical activity. Untreated, it quickly leads to cardiac arrest.

Objective: Cardiovascular Emergencies

Subobjective: Dysrhythmias

23. **C.**

Rationale: PT (prothrombin time) and PTT (partial thromboplastin time) are blood tests that monitor effectiveness of anticoagulant therapy. Hematocrit measures packed RBCs and is not a specific study of anticoagulant effectiveness. HDL and LDL are components of cholesterol measurement. Troponin levels measure myocardial muscle injury.

Objective: Respiratory Emergencies

Subobjective: Pulmonary Embolism

24. **D.**

Rationale: The patient who is diagnosed with disseminated intravascular coagulation (DIC) has both a clotting and bleeding problem. Increased PT/PTT, elevated D-dimer levels, decreased platelets, decreased hemoglobin, and a decreased fibrinogen level are all expected lab values for this patient.

Objective: Medical Emergencies

Subobjective: Blood Dyscrasias

25. **B.**

Rationale: Symptoms of autonomic dysfunction include heart block, bradycardia, hypertension, hypotension, and orthostatic hypotension. Deficits in CN X (vagus nerve) contribute to the development of autonomic dysfunction. Trigeminy, atrial flutter, and tachycardia are not symptoms of autonomic dysfunction.

Objective: Neurological Emergencies

Subobjective: Guillain–Barré Syndrome

26. **C.**

Rationale: Lung tissue disorders include pneumonia and pulmonary edema. Examples of lower airway disorders are bronchiolitis and asthma. An upper airway disorder would be croup, anaphylaxis, or foreign body obstruction. Disordered control of breathing means an irregular, slow breathing pattern with a neurological component, such as a seizure.

Objective: Respiratory Emergencies

Subobjective: Infections

27. **B.**

Rationale: The patient has been playing sports, sweating and replacing lost fluid with only water, which can cause hyponatremia. A loss of sodium will cause neurological effects such as confusion, seizures, and coma. The symptoms are not indicative of a potassium imbalance.

Hyperkalemia would cause thirst and nausea/vomiting.

Objective: Medical Emergencies

Subobjective: Electrolyte/Fluid Imbalance

28. **B.**

    Rationale: A barking cough is a symptom of croup, and nebulized epinephrine is the treatment of choice. IV epinephrine is not indicated in croup; it is more often used in anaphylaxis and resuscitation efforts. Albuterol has a primary effect on lower lung structures and will not improve symptoms of croup. Dexamethasone is indicated for croup but is not the priority intervention.

    Objective: Respiratory Emergencies

    Subobjective: Infections

29. **A.**

    Rationale: Bell's palsy is caused by an inflammation of the seventh cranial nerve and presents with facial paralysis and weakness.

    Objective: Maxillofacial

    Subobjective: Facial Nerve Disorders

30. **B.**

    Rationale: Left-sided heart failure manifestations include pulmonary symptoms such as crackles and dyspnea. Right-sided heart failure causes systemic congestion, leading to hepatomegaly, dependent edema, jugular vein distention, and ascites.

    Objective: Cardiovascular Emergencies

    Subobjective: Heart Failure

31. **A.**

    Rationale: Foreign body infections and cellulitis of surgical hardware sites present with local pain and systemic infectious indicators such as fever, edema, warmth, and elevated WBCs with left shift in neutrophils.

    Objective: Orthopedic

    Subobjective: Foreign Bodies

32. **A.**

    Rationale: Absent or decreased breath sounds are present in a pneumothorax. A nurse would be able to visualize a foreign body on the right side of the chest while doing the initial assessment. Hematoma and pleural effusion are both associated with decreased breath sounds, not with absent sounds.

Objective: Respiratory Emergencies

Subobjective: Pneumothorax

33. **A.**

    Rationale: Warfarin is an anticoagulant commonly prescribed for patients with A-fib. Any anticoagulant must be given cautiously to patients with subarachnoid hemorrhage due to the increased risk of bleeding. Morphine is commonly prescribed for pain, and nimodipine is given to treat or prevent cerebral vasospasm. Stool softeners are given to reduce the need to strain during a bowel movement.

    Objective: Neurological Emergencies

    Subobjective: Trauma

34. **C.**

    Rationale: An uncomfortable feeling of pressure, squeezing, fullness, or pain in the center of the chest is the predominant symptom of a myocardial infarction (MI), particularly in women. Palpitations indicate a dysrhythmia. Edema in the lower extremities is a later sign of cardiac failure. A feeling of nausea is not common with MI.

    Objective: Cardiovascular Emergencies

    Subobjective: Acute Coronary Syndrome

35. **B.**

    Rationale: NPO status is essential for all suspected surgical cases. Elevation is limited with regard to injury. Ice, while therapeutic, would not be a priority intervention.

    Objective: Orthopedic

    Subobjective: Fractures/Dislocations

36. **D.**

    Rationale: Carbamazepine may cause dizziness or drowsiness. The patient should use caution while driving or operating machinery until he understands how the medication will affect him. There is no contraindication to sunlight exposure with this medication. Dietary concerns with carbamazepine are limited to consulting the health care provider before taking with grapefruit juice.

    Objective: Neurological Emergencies

    Subobjective: Seizure Disorders

37. **C.**

Rationale: A Glasgow Coma Scale (GCS) of 7 indicates that the patient is experiencing deficits in eye opening, motor response, and verbal response. As the GCS drops, the patient is less alert and able to follow commands. Patients with a GCS of 7 will require intubation to maintain oxygenation. The lower the GCS, the less likely the patient is to fully recover without permanent deficits. An IV bolus will not negate the need for assisted breathing. This patient will be unable to get up to a chair. As the GCS drops, a nasal cannula becomes ineffective at providing oxygenation.

Objective: Neurological Emergencies

Subobjective: Trauma

38. **D.**

Rationale: A severe headache indicates increased intracranial pressure (ICP), a complication of lumbar puncture. The health care provider should be notified immediately. Other indications of increased ICP are nausea, vomiting, photophobia, and changes in LOC. The patient should be encouraged to increase fluid intake unless contraindicated. The patient will remain flat and on bed rest following the procedure, per agency and health care provider guidelines. Minor pain controlled with analgesics is not a concern but should be monitored for changes.

Objective: Neurological Emergencies

Subobjective: Meningitis

39. **A.**

Rationale: The electrocardiogram (ECG) is most commonly used to initially determine the location of myocardial damage. An echocardiogram is used to view myocardial wall function after a myocardial infarction (MI) has been diagnosed. Cardiac enzymes will aid in diagnosing an MI but will not determine the location. While not performed initially, cardiac catheterization determines coronary artery disease and would suggest the location of myocardial damage.

Objective: Cardiovascular Emergencies

Subobjective: Acute Coronary Syndrome

40. **B.**

Rationale: As Alzheimer's disease progresses, confusion increases. Providing regular toileting can prevent possible falls that result when hurrying to the bathroom to maintain continence. Haloperidol should be used with extreme caution in geriatric patients with Alzheimer's. Restraints can increase confusion in these patients and should be used only per facility guidelines. Offering too many choices can overwhelm the patient and lead to increased confusion and frustration.

Objective: Neurological Emergencies

Subobjective: Alzheimer's Disease/Dementia

41. **A.**

Rationale: N-acetylcysteine is the antidote for acetaminophen toxicity and is administered to patients with hepatotoxic levels of serum acetaminophen levels. Intubation is not indicated, and naloxone is not the correct antidote. Gastric lavage is not indicated in this circumstance.

Objective: Communicable Diseases

Subobjective: Overdose and Ingestion

42. **C.**

Rationale: The patient with emphysema can gain optimal lung expansion by sitting up and leaning forward. Lying in a prone position, flat on the back, or on the side with feet elevated will further potentiate any airway obstruction and effort, exacerbating the problem.

Objective: Respiratory Emergencies

Subobjective: Chronic Obstructive Pulmonary Disease

43. **C.**

Rationale: Validation therapy is used with patients with severe dementia when reality orientation is not appropriate. The nurse may ask the patient what her mother looks like or what she is wearing but does not argue about whether her mother is living. This allows the nurse to acknowledge the patient's concerns while avoiding confrontation or encouraging further belief that her mother is alive. Confrontation may cause the patient with dementia to react inappropriately and is used only when the nurse has established patient trust. Reality orientation works best with patients in the early stages of dementia. Seeking clarification will only cause more confusion because the nurse is asking the patient to explain something, which can lead to patient frustration.

Objective: Neurological Emergencies

Subobjective: Alzheimer's Disease/Dementia

44. **C.**

Rationale: The patient should be thoroughly washed, and all linens and clothing items should be replaced with hospital-provided materials to prevent spread of bedbugs. All home-provided clothing and linens must be double-bagged and either disposed of or placed in a dryer on hot setting for 30 minutes. The presence of bedbugs is not necessarily a sign of abuse or neglect and therefore does not warrant a call to child welfare services. Contact precautions would be most appropriate.

Objective: Environmental

Subobjective: Parasite and Fungal Infestations

45. **D.**

Rationale: A patient with diverticulitis would be expected to have lower abdominal pain with anorexia and fever in addition to an elevated WBC count.

Objective: Gastrointestinal Emergencies

Subobjective: Diverticulitis

46. **B.**

Rationale: An increase in pain with nausea and vomiting are signs that an incarcerated hernia may be causing a bowel obstruction and should be reported immediately. The other findings are expected in a patient with a hernia and do not need to be immediately reported to the health care provider.

Objective: Gastrointestinal Emergencies

Subobjective: Hernia

47. **A.**

Rationale: If the patient has diminished decisional capacity due to a developmental delay, the legal guardian must consent to any intervention for the patient unless there is an emergent issue.

Objective: Professional Issues

Subobjective: System (Patient Consent for Treatment)

48. **C.**

Rationale: This patient is experiencing appendicitis. Pain that is relieved by bending the right hip suggests perforation and peritonitis. The patient would not need an abdominal MRI based on her symptoms. The patient will need surgery, so maintaining NPO status and administering IV fluids are a priority. Morphine will be given for pain.

Objective: Gastrointestinal Emergencies

Subobjective: Acute Abdomen

49. **A.**

Rationale: The first priority for an unresponsive patient in V-fib is performing high-quality CPR. The patient should then be prepared to be defibrillated. Epinephrine should be administered after the patient has been defibrillated at least twice. IV access is not the initial priority.

Objective: Cardiovascular Emergencies

Subobjective: Dysrhythmias

50. **B.**

Rationale: The nursing priority for patients with fistulas is preserving and protecting the skin. The nurse should inspect the skin frequently and assess for any redness, irritation, or broken areas. The skin should remain dry and intact. Antibiotics may be given but are not the first priority. Wound VACs should not be used simply to manage drainage or in patients with increased bleeding risk. Providing a quiet environment is important, but skin integrity is the first priority with this patient.

Objective: Gastrointestinal Emergencies

Subobjective: Inflammatory Bowel Disease

51. **D.**

Rationale: Classic signs of cardiogenic shock include a rapid pulse that weakens; cool, clammy skin; and decreased urine output. Hypotension is another classic sign.

Objective: Cardiovascular Emergencies

Subobjective: Shock

52. **B.**

Rationale: Having a frank, professional conversation regarding chronic pain relief is the nurse's priority. The nurse should not immediately assume the patient is drug-seeking, nor should the nurse ignore the patient's pain complaint.

Objective: Professional Issues

Subobjective:

Patient (Pain Management and Procedural Sedation)

53. D.

Rationale: An avulsion is characterized by the separation of skin from the underlying structures that cannot be approximated.

Objective: Wound

Subobjective: Avulsions

54. C.

Rationale: The priority for this patient is to prepare for surgical removal of the knife, so it should be stabilized with bulky dressings to avoid shifting as the patient is transported. The nurse should never attempt to remove an embedded object in a patient, as this is beyond the scope of practice for nursing. Blood loss may be estimated based on how many dressings or towels are saturated. Next of kin should be notified only after the patient is stabilized.

Objective: Gastrointestinal Emergencies

Subobjective: Abdominal Trauma

55. A.

Rationale: Dysfunction of the renal cells and decreased levels of ADH hormone/vasopressin lead to diuresis, and fluid leakage into the interstitial spaces further contributes to hypovolemia. Shivering and vasoconstriction mask the symptoms of hypovolemia rather than contribute to it. Diaphoresis, dehydration, tachycardia, and tachypnea are all common symptoms of hyperthermia.

Objective: Environmental

Subobjective: Temperature-Related Emergencies

56. A.

Rationale: A sudden, severe onset of testicular pain indicates the possibility of testicular torsion and a stat ultrasound should be ordered to confirm. Epididymitis typically presents gradually with unilateral pain and discharge, and pain is relieved with elevation of the testes. Sudden, severe pain is not an indication of UTI or orchitis.

Objective: Genitourinary

Subobjective: Testicular Torsion

57. B.

Rationale: A purulent vaginal discharge with bilateral pelvic pain and nausea are symptoms of a tubo-ovarian abscess. An ectopic pregnancy would most commonly present with vaginal bleeding, not purulent discharge. A ruptured appendix would typically present as RLQ pain.

Diverticulitis may cause abdominal pain and nausea but not purulent vaginal discharge.

Objective: Gynecological

Subobjective: Infection

58. D.

Rationale: Abdominal cramping with vaginal bleeding and expulsion of tissue are signs of a complete spontaneous abortion. An incomplete spontaneous abortion would have retained tissue. Septic abortions are typically febrile. A threatened abortion may progress to a spontaneous abortion but would not result in passing a large solid tissue clot.

Objective: Obstetrical

Subobjective: Threatened/Spontaneous Abortion

59. C.

Rationale: Corticosteroids will be administered to decrease inflammation of the airways. Albuterol and ipratropium are bronchodilators and do not address the swelling and inflammation caused by croup. Antibiotics are not indicated for croup.

Objective: Respiratory Emergencies

Subobjective: Infections

60. A.

Rationale: The second digit of the nondominant hand is the most common site, as these types of injuries are usually self-inflicted.

Objective: Wound

Subobjective: Injection Injuries

61. A.

Rationale: Mucopurulent discharge, burning, and itching are symptoms of chlamydia. A herpes infection would have lesions. Syphilis typically presents with a small, painless sore. HPV typically presents asymptomatically but may also have warts.

Objective: Gynecological

Subobjective: Infection

62. D.

Rationale: Aspirin is contraindicated for children with varicella because it can lead to Reye's syndrome, a rare form of encephalopathy. Antihistamines, colloidal oatmeal baths, and non-aspirin antipyretics such as acetaminophen are all recommended in-home therapies to relieve symptoms.

Objective: Communicable Diseases

Subobjective: Childhood Diseases

63. B.

Rationale: Current NRP guidelines (2015) recommend 40 – 60 breaths per minute for rescue breathing in the newborn. Rescue breaths at a rate of 12 – 20 are not adequate to provide enough ventilation for the neonate. Inserting an LMA or intubation may be indicated but is not the immediate nursing priority.

Objective: Obstetrical

Subobjective: Neonatal Resuscitation

64. B.

Rationale: As a member of the team the nurse can suggest to the team leader to consider the futility of the resuscitation at that point. The nurse does not have the authority to end the resuscitation and should not advise the patient's parents to make that decision. Ethically, the nurse should speak up if he or she feels that the efforts are futile.

Objective: Professional Issues

Subobjective: Patient (End-of-Life Issues)

65. B.

Rationale: The current (2015) guidelines for neonatal resuscitation recommend epinephrine to be administered at 0.01 – 0.03mg/kg. The other medication dosages are not appropriate as a first-line medication to be administered to a neonate with bradycardia.

Objective: Obstetrical

Subobjective: Neonatal Resuscitation

66. C.

Rationale: Contusions accompanied by the symptoms mentioned should be treated with rest, ice, compression, and elevation. NSAIDs will provide appropriate pain relief; opioid therapy is not indicated for minor contusions.

Objective: Orthopedic

Subobjective: Trauma

67. D.

Rationale: Amitriptyline is a tricyclic antidepressant. This class of drugs has anticholinergic effects, which frequently cause serious side effects. In older, confused patients such as those with Alzheimer's disease, amitriptyline can cause increased confusion, constipation, and urinary retention. Paroxetine and sertraline are SSRIs and may be given to patients with Alzheimer's. Memantine is an NMDA receptor antagonist prescribed to slow the progression of Alzheimer's.

Objective: Neurological Emergencies

Subobjective: Alzheimer's Disease/Dementia

68. B.

Rationale: Adolescent patients presenting with frostbite burns to the roof of the mouth are most likely abusing inhalants, typically in the form of aerosols, glues, paints, and solvents. A hot beverage would not cause the other symptoms, nor would marijuana use. Dry ice would cause tissue injury to the entire mouth.

Objective: Communicable Diseases

Subobjective: Substance Abuse

69. D.

Rationale: The patient should be turned on his side because he may lose consciousness and aspirate. The side-lying position facilitates the drainage of any oral secretions. Padded side rails may be used as part of seizure protocols, but turning the patient on his side is the priority. Tongue blades should never be left at the bedside, as their use can chip teeth, which can be aspirated. Administering IV diazepam should be done only after the patient is turned to his side to avoid aspiration.

Objective: Neurological Emergencies

Subobjective: Seizure Disorders

70. B.

Rationale: The patient has suffered trauma in the motor vehicle crash (MVC). The bright red painless vaginal bleeding is a sign of placenta previa. Abruptio placentae results in painful bleeding that is typically dark red. An ectopic pregnancy and complete abortion would not occur due to an MVC.

Objective: Obstetrical

Subobjective: Placenta Previa

71. A.

Rationale: Abdominal tenderness and dark red vaginal bleeding are signs of abruptio placenta. Placenta previa would present with bright red painless bleeding. Spontaneous abortions typically do not occur after 20 weeks.

Objective: Obstetrical

Subjective: Abruptio Placenta

72. D.

Rationale: Safety is the priority for patients with altered mental status. The nurse should ask if the patient is hearing voices telling him to harm himself or others. Simply saying that no one is there dismisses the patient's feelings. Offering to find a blanket validates the delusion that someone is there. Asking if Martha is staying also prevents reality orientation and may worsen the patient's confusion.

Objective: Psychosocial Emergencies

Subobjective: Psychosis

73. C.

Rationale: A thoracentesis is performed to remove the fluid. A chest tube is used to decompress a hemothorax or pneumothorax and is not indicated in the presence of pleural effusion. A pericardial window is used to drain excess fluid from the pericardium, not the pleural space.

Objective: Respiratory Emergencies

Subobjective: Plural Effusion

74. B.

Rationale: Esophageal varices can lead to death via hemorrhage. Octreotide is a vasoconstrictor used to control bleeding before performing endoscopy. Phenytoin is an anticonvulsant, levofloxacin is an antibiotic, and pantoprazole is a proton pump inhibitor; none of these are indicated at this time.

Objective: Gastrointestinal Emergencies

Subobjective: Esophageal Varices

75. D.

Rationale: "You're feeling lost since your mother died," uses the therapeutic technique of restating. The nurse repeats the patient's words back to her. This therapeutic communication technique allows the patient to verify that the nurse understood the patient and allows for clarification if needed. It also encourages the patient to continue. Telling the patient that she will feel better in time minimizes the patient's feelings and sounds uncaring. Telling the patient to join a grief support group forces the nurse's decision onto the patient. Stating shared feelings takes the focus from the patient to the nurse.

Objective: Psychosocial Emergencies

Subobjective: Depression

76. D.

Rationale: The symptoms indicate right-sided myocardial infarction (MI), so IV fluids are the priority treatment for this patient. When treating patients with right ventricular infarction, nitrates, diuretics, and morphine are to be avoided due to their pre-load-reducing effects.

Objective: Cardiac Emergencies

Subobjective: Acute Coronary Syndromes

77. C.

Rationale: The symptoms are characteristic of meningococcal meningitis, which is commonly contracted in crowded living spaces such as college dorms. Influenza is characterized by upper-respiratory symptoms; scabies is a dermal infection; and pertussis is a respiratory illness.

Objective: Communicable Diseases

Subobjective: Childhood Diseases

78. D.

Rationale: Endoscopic ligation is indicated for *posterior* epistaxis stemming from the ethmoid or sphenopalatine arteries. Kiesselbach's plexus is the most common site of *anterior* epistaxis that responds to conventional treatments.

Objective: Maxillofacial

Subobjective: Epistaxis

79. B.

Rationale: The patient with adrenal hypofunction should not be on a sodium-restrictive diet, as it may lead to an adrenal crisis. Peripheral blood draws, glucose monitoring, and hydrocortisone therapy are all appropriate for adrenal insufficiency.

Objective: Medical Emergencies

Subobjective: Endocrine Conditions

80. B.

Rationale: The patient has had nausea and vomiting, which can cause hypokalemia. A U wave can be noted on an ECG or cardiac monitor. Hyperkalemia would show peaked T waves. Hypercalcemia may produce a shortened QT interval, and hypocalcemia may show QT prolongation.

Objective: Medical Emergencies

Subobjective: Electrolyte/Fluid Imbalance

81. **A.**

Rationale: Chain of custody is the concept of limiting the number of people handling and collecting evidence after a crime is committed. Nurses caring for patients and handling evidence should use local official documents to demonstrate the chain of custody for evidence and to document when it is given to authorities.

Objective: Professional Issues

Subobjective: Patient (Forensic Evidence Collection)

82. **C.**

Rationale: The patient has a pneumothorax and will need a chest tube. Chest compressions are indicated only for cardiac arrest. Thoracotomy is done when there is severe trauma and impending or present cardiac arrest and is the final effort made to sustain life; it is associated with a low rate of successful outcomes. Endotracheal intubation is not indicated if the patient is able to protect his own airway, as is evidenced by his ability to communicate verbally.

Objective: Respiratory Emergencies

Subobjective: Pneumothorax

83. **C.**

Rationale: Patients with hyperventilation syndrome will present with similar signs and symptoms as pulmonary emboli. Patients with a pneumothorax will present with absent breath sounds on the side of the injury, anxiety, and pain on inspiration. Pneumonia is characterized by fever, malaise, and crackles at the base of the lungs.

Objective: Respiratory Emergencies

Subobjective: Pulmonary Embolus

84. **A.**

Rationale: Antipsychotics are used to treat psychotic symptoms such as hallucinations, paranoia, and delusions. They carry an increased risk of mortality, primarily from cardiovascular complications. A cardiac workup identifies any risk factors that would be a contraindication to antipsychotics. A comprehensive metabolic panel (CMP), creatinine clearance, and a CBC do not address the underlying risk of cardiovascular complications.

Objective: Psychosocial Emergencies

Subobjective: Psychosis

85. **C.**

Rationale: The nurse should assign a sitter because the patient's safety is more important than his right to refuse care. Placing the patient in restraints does not guarantee his safety and may escalate the situation. If the patient manages to get out of the restraints, he might hang himself with them. Having security sit outside the door does not provide direct observation of the patient and uses up a limited resource of the facility. Allowing the patient to leave against medical advice (AMA) leaves the nurse and the facility vulnerable to legal action if he commits suicide after leaving.

Objective: Psychosocial Emergencies

Subobjective: Suicidal Ideation

86. **A.**

Rationale: Abnormalities in magnesium levels may put the patient at risk for ventricular dysrhythmia. A hypomagnesemia level of 0.8 mEq/L would be of concern (normal range is 1.5 – 2.5 mEq/L). The other values are within normal ranges.

Objective: Cardiovascular Emergencies

Subobjective: Dysrhythmias

87. **D.**

Rationale: The patient is experiencing an unstable supraventricular tachycardia (SVT) with BP of 70/42 mm Hg and requires immediate synchronized cardioversion. Defibrillation is not indicated because the patient is awake and has an organized heart rhythm. Adenosine can be used in patients with stable SVT; however, this patient is not stable. Amiodarone is not indicated for unstable patients in SVT.

Objective: Cardiovascular Emergencies

Subobjective: Dysrhythmias

88. **A.**

Rationale: The drug of choice for supraventricular tachycardia (SVT) is adenosine. The first dose of 6 mg has already been given, so the next appropriate dose would be 12 mg. The other options are not the next appropriate intervention for a patient in SVT.

Objective: Cardiovascular Emergencies

Subobjective: Dysrhythmias

89. A.

Rationale: The patient experiencing a sickle cell crisis needs fluid resuscitation with crystalloid solutions and the administration of warmed RBCs. Whole blood contains additional components such as plasma or platelets, which are not needed. Fresh frozen plasma and cryoprecipitate are not indicated for sickle cell crisis.

Objective: Medical Emergencies

Subobjective: Blood Dyscrasias

90. B.

Rationale: The goal for pulse oximetry readings is 94% – 99%. The nurse should apply supplemental oxygen for an SpO_2 below 94%. Albuterol and dexamethasone are appropriate for asthma but are not the priority intervention. Endotracheal intubation is needed only if a patient is unable to maintain their airway.

Objective: Respiratory Emergencies

Subobjective: Asthma

91. B.

Rationale: Rhabdomyolysis is characterized by the breakdown of skeletal muscle with the release of myoglobin and other intercellular proteins and electrolytes into the circulation. The presence of myoglobin produces heme-positive results in the urinalysis.

Objective: Orthopedic

Subobjective: Trauma

92. D.

Rationale: The sharp, tearing knifelike substernal chest pain with no relief from morphine is a hallmark sign of an aortic dissection. Pneumonia presents with pain related to coughing. Pain from a myocardial infarction (MI) or pericarditis would likely be relieved with doses of morphine sulfate.

Objective: Cardiovascular Emergencies

Subobjective: Aneurysm/Dissection

93. B.

Rationale: Captopril is an ACE inhibitor, which can cause hyperkalemia. Bumetanide and furosemide are diuretics, which would cause hypokalemia. Digoxin is an antidysrhythmic and can also cause hypokalemia.

Objective: Medical Emergencies

Subobjective: Electrolyte/Fluid Imbalance

94. C.

Rationale: Patients with idiopathic thrombocytopenic purpura (ITP) have decreased platelet production, so platelets are the expected treatment. The other options are not indicated for this condition.

Objective: Medical Emergencies

Subobjective: Blood Dyscrasias

95. C.

Rationale: Vasospastic disorders such as Raynaud's phenomena and migraine headaches are associated with variant (Prinzmetal's) angina.

Objective: Cardiac Emergencies

Subobjective: Chronic Stable Angina Pectoris

96. B.

Rationale: Hyperosmolar hyperglycemic state (HHS) is often caused by dehydration, especially in patients over 65. Inadequate glucose monitoring and medication noncompliance are not the most common causes of HHS. A breakdown of ketones causing ketoacidosis would be found in diabetic ketoacidosis (DKA).

Objective: Medical Emergencies

Subobjective: Endocrine Conditions

97. C.

Rationale: Fluoxetine is given cautiously to patients with glaucoma, due to the anticholinergic side effects. There are no current indications that this medication causes side effects with arthritis, migraines, or appendicitis.

Objective: Psychosocial Emergencies

Subobjective: Depression

98. D.

Rationale: Throbbing fingers or toes after exercise accompanied with thin, shiny skin and thick fingernails are symptoms of peripheral vascular disease. Acute occlusion would present with pain and cyanosis distal to the occlusion. Venous thrombosis occurs more often in the lower extremities, and there is no information suggesting arterial injury.

Objective: Cardiovascular Emergencies

Subobjective: Peripheral Vascular Disease

99. C.

Rationale: Insulin administration shifts potassium into the cells causing hypokalemia, so fluids with potassium are indicated for this patient. The other fluids are not indicated for this patient.

Objective: Medical Emergencies

Subobjective: Endocrine Conditions

100. A.

Rationale: Propylthiouracil (PTU) is the drug of choice in treating thyroid storm, as it inhibits the synthesis of thyroxine. Epinephrine and atropine are contraindicated for thyroid storm, as these patients already have a dangerously high heart rate. Levothyroxine would be indicated for myxedema coma.

Objective: Medical Emergencies

Subobjective: Endocrine Conditions

101. C.

Rationale: Status epilepticus occurs when a person experiences a seizure that lasts more than 5 minutes or has repeated episodes over 30 minutes. This is a medical emergency, as death can result if seizures last more than 10 minutes. Causes of status epilepticus include alcohol or drug withdrawal, suddenly stopping antiseizure medications, head trauma, and infection. Atonic seizures occur when the patient has a sudden loss of muscle tone for a few seconds, followed by postictal confusion. Tonic–clonic (grand mal) seizures last for only a few minutes. With a simple partial seizure, the patient remains conscious during the episode, which may be preceded by auras. Autonomic changes may occur, such as heart rate changes and epigastric discomfort.

Objective: Neurological Emergencies

Subobjective: Seizure Disorders

102. B.

Rationale: Risk factors for pancreatitis include alcohol abuse, peptic ulcer disease, renal failure, vascular disorders, hyperlipidemia, and hyperparathyroidism. Patients often find relief in the fetal position, while the supine position worsens pain. The pain is severe and sudden and feels intense and boring, as if it is going through the body. Pain occurs in the mid-epigastric area or left upper quadrant. Pain can radiate to the left flank, the left shoulder, or the back.

Objective: Gastrointestinal Emergencies

Subobjective: Pancreatitis

103. B.

Rationale: A family member at the bedside for resuscitation has been demonstrated in the evidence as a preference for patients and families and should be offered when possible and appropriate. Family members should be present only if they are not disruptive to patient care.

104. A.

Rationale: When an organ donor patient dies in the ED the nurse should first contact the organ procurement organization because of time sensitivity. Life-supporting interventions such as ventilators and medications should be continued until the organ procurement agency arrives. Postmortem care and completing the death certificate can be performed after organ procurement has taken place.

Objective: Professional Issues

Subobjective: Patient (End-of-Life Issues)

105. B.

Rationale: An elevation in serum lactate level will conclude the diagnosis of sepsis. The WBC count and neutrophil count would be increased. RBCs do not give adequate information to suspect sepsis.

Objective: Medical Emergencies

Subobjective: Sepsis and Septic Shock

106. C.

Rationale: The patient will be involuntarily committed because she is a threat to her own safety. She has not committed a crime. She will not be admitted voluntarily because she did not come to the hospital of her own volition.

Objective: Professional Issues

Subobjective: Patient (Transitions of Care)

107. D.

Rationale: The patient is in acidosis and has Kussmaul respirations, which are indicative of diabetic ketoacidosis (DKA). Myxedema coma and pheochromocytoma would not cause these symptoms. Hyperosmolar hyperglycemic state (HHS) normally causes higher blood sugar levels and does not present in acidosis.

Objective: Medical Emergencies

Subobjective: Endocrine Conditions

108. B.

Rationale: The Glasgow Coma Scale (GCS) is calculated as follows: opening eyes to sound (3), localizing pain (5), and making incoherent sounds (2) gives a GCS score of 10.

Objective: Neurological Emergencies

Subobjective: Trauma

109. A.

Rationale: The patient is showing signs of peritonsillar abscess. Peritonsillar abscess is an emergent condition that occurs from the accumulation of purulent exudate between the tonsillar capsule and the pharyngeal constrictor muscle. Patchy tonsillar exudate, petechiae, and lymphedema are common findings with viral and bacterial strep throat infections.

Objective: Maxillofacial

Subobjective: Peritonsillar Abscess

110. C.

Rationale: Foods high in lactose may be poorly tolerated by patients with ulcerative colitis (UC) and should be limited or avoided. High-fiber foods can aggravate GI symptoms in some patients and should be avoided. Caffeine is a stimulant that can increase cramping and diarrhea. Dried fruit stimulates the GI tract and can exacerbate symptoms.

Objective: Gastrointestinal Emergencies

Subobjective: Inflammatory Bowel Disease

111. C.

Rationale: A sudden sharp pain in the pelvic region associated with sexual intercourse and no vaginal discharge is common with an ovarian cyst rupture. An ectopic pregnancy does not typically present with sudden pain, and there is usually vaginal bleeding. A ruptured appendix will cause constant pain to the RLQ and commonly causes a fever. The symptoms are not indicative of an STD.

Objective: Gynecological

Subobjective: Ovarian Cyst

112. B.

Rationale: Dehydration requires an isotonic crystalloid solution, such as normal saline or lactated Ringer's, which will evenly distribute between the intravascular space and cells. Hypertonic solutions pull water from cells into the intravascular space, and hypotonic solutions move fluid from the intravascular space into the cells.

Colloid solutions, such as albumin, draw fluid into intravascular compartments and would not be appropriate for this patient.

Objective: Medical Emergencies

Subobjective: Electrolyte/Fluid Imbalance

113. C.

Rationale: A history of hypertension will cause an increase in afterload. Diabetes will cause complications with microvascular disease, leading to poor cardiac function. Endocrine disorders will cause an increase in cardiac workload. Marfan syndrome causes the cardiac muscle to stretch and weaken.

Objective: Cardiac Emergencies

Subobjective: Heart Failure

114. D.

Rationale: Patients with subarachnoid hemorrhage commonly describe having the "worst headache of my life." Nausea and vomiting, not food cravings, may occur. There is no rash associated with subarachnoid hemorrhage. Battle's sign is a characteristic symptom of basilar skull fracture.

Objective: Neurological Emergencies

Subobjective: Trauma

115. B.

Rationale: The signs and symptoms of pelvic inflammatory disease are lower abdominal pain that worsens with movement, a temperature greater than 101.3°F (38.5°C), tachycardia, and non-malodorous vaginal discharge. Appendicitis does not cause vaginal discharge. Ectopic pregnancy typically causes vaginal bleeding. Most STIs present with malodorous discharge and do not cause fever and tachycardia.

Objective: Gynecological

Subobjective: Infection

116. C.

Rationale: Several of the medications used to treat MS are immunosuppressants; therefore, the patient is more susceptible to infection while taking them. Patients should avoid crowds and anyone who appears to have an infection, such as the flu. Alternating an eye patch from one eye to the other every few hours can relieve diplopia. Patients with MS have alterations in mobility, and clearing walking paths in the home makes it safer to ambulate, especially with a walker or cane. If the patient suspects infection, he or she should notify the health care provider immediately.

Objective: Neurological Emergencies

Subobjective: Chronic Neurological Disorders

117. **C.**

Rationale: Penicillin V potassium for antibiotic therapy is indicated for the treatment of dental abscesses, a condition indicated by this patient's symptoms. Sodium fluoride drops are a supplement for children, nystatin is used to treat oral candida albicans infections, and saliva substitute is a rinse for dry mouth.

Objective: Maxillofacial

Subobjective: Dental Conditions

118. **C.**

Rationale: Morphine sulfate is the analgesic of choice in acute coronary syndrome (ACS): it provides analgesic and sedation and also decreases preload and afterload. Morphine is administered to relieve pain as well as to decrease pain-related anxiety that can further exacerbate the symptoms of the myocardial infarction (MI). Meperidine is not indicated for use in MI. Hydromorphone is more appropriate for patients with no cardiac compromise, and acetaminophen is not indicated in MI.

Objective: Cardiovascular Emergencies

Subobjective: Acute Coronary Syndrome

119. **A.**

Rationale: HIV patients with a fever are considered emergent, and a septic workup is expected. After drawing blood cultures, antibiotics should be the priority intervention. Acetaminophen may be administered but is not the priority. Giving the patient antivirals after she has been noncompliant is not a priority. She does not need a blood transfusion.

Objective: Medical Emergencies

Subobjective: Immunocompromised

120. **C.**

Rationale: Late signs of increased intracranial pressure (ICP) include dilated or pinpoint pupils that are sluggish or nonreactive to light. Headache, restlessness, and decreasing LOC are early signs of increased ICP.

Objective: Neurological Emergencies

Subobjective: Increased Intracranial Pressure (ICP)

121. **A.**

Rationale: The child should remain with the parent in an upright position. Taking the child from the parent could cause anxiety and crying and worsen the respiratory distress.

Objective: Respiratory Emergencies

Subobjective: Infections

122. **A.**

Rationale: Complications of ulcerative colitis (UC) include hemorrhage and nutritional deficiencies. Patients may have up to 10 – 20 bloody, liquid stools per day. Loose, non-bloody stools and fistulas are more common in patients with Crohn's disease. Surgery is rarely required for these symptoms.

Objective: Gastrointestinal Emergencies

Subobjective: Inflammatory Bowel Disease

123. **B.**

Rationale: Trigeminal neuralgia pain has an abrupt onset, is unilateral along the branch of the fifth cranial nerve, and causes hemifacial spasms.

Objective: Maxillofacial

Subobjective: Facial Nerve Disorders

124. **C.**

Rationale: The patient is experiencing symptoms of pulmonary edema, a complication of left-sided heart failure. Coagulation is not a secondary effect of myocardial infarction (MI). Pneumonia is not generally related to post–MI concerns. A ruptured ventricle would present symptoms closer to the time of injury.

Objective: Cardiovascular Emergencies

Subobjective: Heart Failure and Cardiogenic Pulmonary Edema

125. **B.**

Rationale: Advance directives must be valid, up to date, and documented before they can be honored in the ED. The nurse can document the patient's wishes, but it is not official until the paperwork is present. The physician does not make that decision, and with the correct documentation, EDs will honor advance directives.

Objective: Professional Issues

Subobjective: Patient (End-of-Life Issues)

126. **D.**

Rationale: A pharmacist would not be consulted in this situation. Other members of the team may include ED physicians, social workers, and hospital religious team members.

Objective: Professional Issues

Subobjective: Patient (End-of-Life Issues)

127. **C.**

Rationale: Instruct the parent to perform oral positive pressure by sealing his or her mouth securely over the child's mouth and providing a short, sharp puff of air while simultaneously occluding the unaffected nostril.

Objective: Maxillofacial

Subobjective: Foreign Bodies

128. **A.**

Rationale: The patient's ammonia level and ALT are elevated, which is expected with cirrhosis. Lactulose is given to lower ammonia levels in patients with cirrhosis. Bisacodyl is a laxative and is not indicated for this patient. Mesalamine is an anti-inflammatory given for ulcerative colitis. The patient's blood glucose is not elevated enough to require 2 units of insulin.

Objective: Gastrointestinal Emergencies

Subobjective: Cirrhosis

129. **C.**

Rationale: Patching the affected eye decreases oxygen delivery to the cornea, delays wound healing, and creates an environment that increases the risk for infection.

Objective: Ocular

Subobjective: Abrasions

130. **D.**

Rationale: When a patient is experiencing hallucinations, the nurse should acknowledge the patient's fear but reinforce reality. Telling the patient that it is the wrinkles in the blanket dismisses the patient's fear and does not reorient the patient. Offering to move the patient to another room accepts the snakes as real and does not help the patient with reality. Offering to call maintenance reinforces the patient's belief that the snakes are real.

Objective: Psychosocial Emergencies

Subobjective: Psychosis

131. **D.**

Rationale: Isocarboxazid and other MAOIs should not be taken with rasagiline mesylate due to the risk of increased blood pressure and hypertensive crisis. The other medications are not contraindicated for this patient: baclofen relieves muscle spasms, benztropine is an older drug that treats severe motor symptoms such as rigidity and tremors, and amantadine is an antiviral drug often prescribed with carbidopa and levodopa to reduce dyskinesias.

Objective: Neurological Emergencies

Subobjective: Chronic Neurological Disorders

132. **A.**

Rationale: Herpes zoster infection of the facial nerves commonly involves the eyelid and surrounding structures. Treatment is palliative, using antiviral medications such as acyclovir.

Objective: Ocular

Subobjective: Infections

133. **C.**

Rationale: Patients with ulcerative keratitis MUST NOT use contact lenses until the infection has resolved and been cleared by an ophthalmologist. The patient should complete the full course of prescribed antibiotics. Not all ulcers are contagious, so she could safely return to work after 24 hours of antibiotic use.

Objective: Ocular

Subobjective: Ulcerations/Keratitis

134. **D.**

Rationale: These ABGs indicate acute respiratory acidosis. Common signs of respiratory acidosis include hypoventilation with hypoxia, disorientation, and dizziness. Untreated respiratory acidosis can progress to ventricular fibrillation, hypotension, seizures, and coma. Deep, rapid respirations and nausea and vomiting are signs of metabolic acidosis. Chest pain is not a symptom of respiratory acidosis.

Objective: Respiratory Emergencies

Subobjective: Chronic Obstructive Pulmonary Disorder

135. **A.**

Rationale: Iritis is treated with topical mydriatic ophthalmic drops to dilate the pupil, topical corticosteroids to reduce inflammation, and referral to ophthalmology within 24 hours.

Objective: Ocular

Subobjective: Infections

136. D.

Rationale: Clinical open globe rupture features include afferent pupillary defect, impaired visual acuity, gross deformity of the eye, and prolapsing uvea.

Objective: Ocular

Subobjective: Trauma

137. A.

Rationale: A commercially available tourniquet at least 2 inches wide with a windlass or ratcheting device is recommended for both prehospital and in-hospital use. The nurse should never remove a tourniquet without team support to control hemorrhagic bleeding. Assessment occurs in 2-hour intervals.

Objective: Orthopedic

Subobjective: Amputation

138. D.

Rationale: Dopamine (Intropin) is a positive inotrope, which will increase cardiac contractility and cardiac output, decrease the myocardial workload, and improve myocardial oxygen delivery.

Objective: Cardiovascular Emergencies

Subobjective: Heart Failure

139. D.

Rationale: Only the CT angiography will confirm the diagnosis. D-dimer may be increased in the presence of pulmonary embolism (PE) but is not a stand-alone indicator for definitive diagnosis. A chest X-ray will rule out other disease processes but does not rule in a PE. Fibrin split products are measured in the presence of disseminated intravascular coagulation and are not relevant for the concern of PE.

Objective: Respiratory Emergencies

Subobjective: Pulmonary Embolism

140. B.

Rationale: When caring for mentally unstable or possibly violent patients, staff safety is the primary concern. The nurse should avoid getting blocked into a corner between the patient and the door. If possible, the patient should be in a room near the nurses' station, and the nurse should notify someone before entering the room. Bringing another nurse or patient care technician can also maintain safety. All patients should be treated with courtesy and respect, especially someone who may be prone to paranoia. It may be necessary to observe the patient closely for "cheeking" pills instead of swallowing them. Some medications may be ordered in IV form to ensure that the patient receives the medication if he has surreptitiously avoided swallowing pills in the past. Always ask permission before touching or approaching the patient to avoid startling him. If the patient refuses medications or blood draws, do not argue. Chart the refusal in the medical record and notify the health care provider.

Objective: Psychosocial Emergencies

Subobjective: Aggressive/Violent Behavior

141. D.

Rationale: Costochondritis occurs from localized inflammation of the joints attaching the ribs to the sternum and most commonly presents in females ages 12 to 14.

Objective: Orthopedic

Subobjective: Costochondritis

142. C.

Rationale: Gouty arthritis characteristically occurs in patients with hyperuricemia, which causes high levels of uric acid in the blood from breakdown of purines. Hyperammonemia is the presence of an excess of ammonia in the blood. Hyperbilirubinemia is too much bilirubin in the blood. Hyperhomocysteinemia is a marker for the development of heart disease.

Objective: Orthopedic

Subobjective: Inflammatory Conditions

143. A.

Rationale: In a flail chest there is asymmetrical movement of the chest wall. Ribs are completely broken and cause abnormal movement of the chest wall. As the patient breathes in, the flail segment will sink in; as the patient breathes out, the segment will bulge outward.

Objective: Respiratory Emergencies

Subobjective: Trauma

144. B.

Rationale: Avulsed primary teeth are not replanted because of the potential for subsequent damage to the developing permanent tooth and the increased frequency of pulpal necrosis. Best initial management would be to repair the lacerations.

Objective: Maxillofacial

Subobjective: Dental Conditions

145. C.

Rationale: Nonstick adherent dressing such as a Band-Aid or Telfa pad is the appropriate choice.

Objective: Wound

Subobjective: Abrasions

146. B.

Rationale: There should be a high index of suspicion that the patient experienced an inhalation injury, and measures should be taken to protect her airway. Burns and trauma are secondary concerns to airway compromise. Soot at the mouth opening suggests smoke inhalation, not foreign body ingestion.

Objective: Respiratory Emergencies

Subobjective: Inhalation Injuries

147. C.

Rationale: Dimming lights or providing a blindfold are contraindicated, as low lighting will increase pupillary size, creating an increase in intraocular pressure. Pupil size should remain constricted through use of bright lighting and miotic ophthalmic drops.

Objective: Ocular

Subobjective: Glaucoma

148. B.

Rationale: Chest pain can occur with the first dose of sumatriptan and should be reported immediately. Sumatriptan may not be safe for pregnant women, so the patient should be coached on using an effective birth control method while taking it. Most triptans are contraindicated with hypertension and would not be prescribed if the patient is taking antihypertensives due to the risk of coronary vasospasm. The medication should be taken as soon as the first symptoms of migraine appear.

Objective: Neurological Emergencies

Subobjective: Headache

149. A.

Rationale: The typical chest radiography for a patient with adult respiratory distress syndrome

(ARDS) is bilateral, diffuse white infiltrates without cardiomegaly. Options C and D show results for abnormal heart tissue but not for lung tissue and do not give any information about infiltrates.

Objective: Respiratory Emergencies

Subobjective: Respiratory Distress Syndrome

150. B.

Rationale: Many opioid substances are commonly injected, resulting in abscess formation from use of non-sterile equipment and aseptic technique. Cocaine, amphetamines, and other substances may also be injected. Alcohol, benzodiazepine, and tetrahydrocannabinol use may be co-occurring in the patient, but these substances are not commonly injected.

Objective: Wound

Subobjective: Infections

151. C.

Rationale: The patient is hypotensive, hypothermic, and bradycardic. He has ingested thyroid replacement medications and sedatives, which can lead to a myxedema coma. The symptoms are not indicative of an allergic reaction or an acute stroke. A thyroid storm would show increased heart rate, temperature, and blood pressure.

Objective: Medical Emergencies

Subobjective: Endocrine Conditions

152. D.

Rationale: Epinephrine is never used for lacerations of the fingers, toes, face, or penis.

Objective: Wound

Subobjective: Lacerations

153. C.

Rationale: Post-exposure prophylaxis in a patient who has not been vaccinated must consist of both immunoglobin and vaccine therapy. While up-to-date tetanus immunization should be considered, it is a targeted vaccine against infection by *Clostridium tetani*.

Objective: Environmental

Subobjective: Vector-Borne Illnesses

154. D.

Rationale: The child is presenting with signs of asthma exacerbation. Symptoms of foreign body aspiration are consistent with acute airway obstruction to include respiratory distress and drooling. Pneumonitis would present with chest pain and dyspnea but not these acute symptoms. Pneumonia is characterized with crackles in the lower lobes and decreased oxygen saturation.

Objective: Respiratory Emergencies

Subobjective: Asthma

155. **A.**

Rationale: The patient will need epinephrine administered immediately. Most anaphylactic deaths occur due to a delay in epinephrine administration. Diphenhydramine and Solu-Medrol are indicated for minor allergic reactions. Theophylline is typically used to treat asthma and is not indicated for anaphylaxis.

Objective: Medical Emergencies

Subobjective: Allergic Reactions and Anaphylaxis

156. **B.**

Rationale: Hyperbaric oxygen is used to treat severe carbon monoxide toxicity. Hydroxocobalamin is a cyanide-binding agent. *N*-acetylcysteine restores depleted hepatic glutathione, reversing effects of acetaminophen toxicity. Sodium bicarbonate is standard treatment for salicylate toxicity.

Objective: Environmental

Subobjective: Chemical Exposure

157. **C.**

Rationale: Patients presenting with vague neurological symptoms may be difficult to diagnose. The history and information leading up to presentation in the department is vital in determining differential diagnoses. This patient is not presenting with stroke-like symptoms. The symptoms are similar to those of a migraine; however, the history makes carbon monoxide poisoning more likely. The patient is not demonstrating stroke or allergic reaction symptoms.

Objective: Toxicology

Subobjective: Carbon Monoxide

158. **C.**

Rationale: Calcium gluconate is administered to the patient with hyperkalemia for cardiac and neuromuscular protection. Aspirin is used for acute coronary syndrome but would not be a first-line drug for this condition. Insulin and dextrose may be given to lower potassium levels but do not function to protect cardiac status. Digoxin is an antidysrhythmic and is not indicated for hyperkalemia.

Objective: Medical Emergencies

Subobjective: Renal Failure

159. **C.**

Rationale: Monitoring neurological status is the most important nursing intervention for patients with meningitis. Deficits of cranial nerve VI prevent lateral eye movement, which is an indicator of hydrocephalus. Other indicators of hydrocephalus include urinary incontinence and signs of increased intracranial pressure (ICP). Declining LOC is the first sign of increased ICP, and the nurse must be sensitive to even small changes in LOC. The other findings do not indicate increasing ICP.

Objective: Neurological Emergencies

Subobjective: Increased Intracranial Pressure (ICP)

160. **B.**

Rationale: Patients with diverticular disease should remain on clear liquids until pain has subsided. For maintenance, they will need to eat 25 to 35 grams of fiber daily to provide bulk to the stool. Patients should avoid high-sodium foods and alcohol, which irritates the bowel. Strawberries contain seeds that may block a diverticulum and should be avoided, along with nuts, corn, popcorn, and tomatoes.

Objective: Gastrointestinal Emergencies

Subobjective: Diverticulitis

161. **D.**

Rationale: Keraunoparalysis is a condition specific to lightning strikes, resulting from vasoconstriction in the tissues surrounding entry and exit points. Ascending paralysis is a common finding in Guillain–Barré syndrome. Bell's palsy and tic douloureux are both facial nerve disorders.

Objective: Environmental

Subobjective: Electrical Injuries

162. **B.**

Rationale: The patient's last drink is important to determine the possibility of withdrawal or delirium tremens. The other questions are relevant but are not the priority based on the patient's presentation.

Objective: Communicable Diseases

Subobjective: Withdrawal Syndrome

163. C.

Rationale: Octreotide is used for overdoses refractory to glucose administration. It stimulates the release of insulin from the beta islet cells of the pancreas. Flumazenil is the antidote for benzodiazepine overdose. Acetylcysteine is used for acetaminophen overdose, and methylene blue is used for nitrites and anesthetics overdose.

Objective: Communicable Diseases

Subobjective: Overdose and Ingestion

164. B.

Rationale: Tuberculosis is characterized by a cough lasting 2 – 3 weeks or more, fever, chills, night sweats, and fatigue. The recent travel to a developing country is a concern for potential infectious disease. The other conditions have similar symptoms, but the travel and chronic cough indicate strong concern for pulmonary tuberculosis.

Objective: Communicable Diseases

Subobjective: Tuberculosis

165. B.

Rationale: Calcium channel blockers can cause symptoms in children with doses as low as 1 tablet. Rapid deterioration may occur if the tablets are short acting. A 5-year-old may not accurately count or recollect the number of tablets consumed. A referral to child protective services should be made if there is a reasonable suspicion for the need but is not a priority intervention. Oxygen should be provided only if pulse oximetry is less than 92%.

Objective: Communicable Diseases

Subobjective: Overdose and Ingestion

166. B.

Rationale: People who chronically abuse alcohol are deficient in thiamine and are given IV thiamine. Naloxone blocks opioid receptors and is given for opioid overdose. Flumazenil is a benzodiazepine receptor antagonist and is given for benzodiazepine overdose. Vitamin K is given for warfarin overdose.

Objective: Communicable Diseases

Subobjective: Substance Abuse

167. C.

Rationale: The rash, conjunctivitis, and cough are indicative of measles, and the patient's vaccination status makes this diagnosis even more likely. Varicella is characterized by vesicular rash on the trunk and face; mumps, by nonspecific respiratory symptoms and edema in the parotid gland; and pertussis is a respiratory disease with a specific "whoop"-sounding cough.

Objective: Communicable Diseases

Subobjective: Childhood Diseases

168. A.

Rationale: Herpes zoster, also known as shingles, is caused by the reactivation of the dormant varicella virus. It can occur several times over the lifetime of a patient who has had an initial varicella infection. The varicella vaccine is not known to cause herpes zoster. Herpes zoster can be spread by contact with the rash; someone who has never had varicella may contract it from contact with a herpes zoster rash. The zoster vaccine may prevent a second or third outbreak in patients who have had active herpes zoster.

Objective: Communicable Diseases

Subobjective: Herpes Zoster

169. A.

Rationale: A pseudomembrane, or thick gray membrane, covering the tonsils, the pharynx, and sometimes the larynx is characteristic of diphtheria infection. Patients with diphtheria may have a low-grade fever; they will not have a macular rash or headache.

Objective: Communicable Diseases

Subobjective: Childhood Diseases

170. C.

Rationale: The nurse demonstrates personal insight that further help is needed via the Critical Incident Stress Management (CISM) system. CISM does not require or recommend that nurses needing debriefing or assistance meet with managers specifically about the event or experience. The nurse should not depart the debriefing before it is complete, and future debrief sessions may or may not occur. Scheduling appointments is a concrete action that demonstrates the nurse's effective participation.

Objective: Professional Issues

Subobjective: Nurse (Critical Incident Stress Management)

171. B.

Rationale: Participation and engagement in Evidence-Based Practice (EBP) projects supports an environment of quality and safe care using up-to-date evidence and practices that have been thoroughly researched. Reading research articles is important, but the data must be synthesized through formal processes to implement evidence into practice.

Objective: Professional Issues

Subobjective: Nurse (Evidence-Based Practice)

172. D.

Rationale: Patient income is not directly relevant to transitions of care and is not appropriate for ED nurses to ask about when managing care transitions. Safety, community partnerships, and accessibility of services are all appropriate considerations.

Objective: Professional Issues

Subobjective: Patient (Transitions of Care)

173. D.

Rationale: The current (2015) AHA and NRP guidelines for newborn resuscitation is 3 compressions to 1 ventilation. A ratio of 30:2 is appropriate for all adults or a single rescuer infant/child; a ratio of 15:2 is appropriate for 2 rescuers with children and infants. A ratio of 15:1 is not recommended for anyone.

Objective: Obstetrical

Subobjective: Neonatal Resuscitation

174. D.

Rationale: A Foley catheter is not necessary to decompress the bladder in this patient. Typically, these patients are eligible for eye donation, and the head should be at 20 degrees, with artificial tears or saline in the eyes to preserve the tissue. Tape should be used if eyes do not close after death.

Objective: Professional Issues

Subobjective: Patient (End-of-Life Issues)

175. B.

Rationale: Annular lesions with raised borders and cleared central areas of the rash indicate ringworm. Scabies are characterized by red pruritic rashes, and cellulitis and impetigo do not present in this way.

Objective: Environmental

Subobjective: Parasite and Fungal Infestations

Follow the link below to take your SECOND CEN practice test:

www.triviumtestprep.com/cen-online-resources

Made in the USA
Coppell, TX
22 October 2020